普通高等教育“十一五”国家级规划教材

全国高等医药院校药学类专业第二轮实验双语教材

生物药剂学实验与指导

（第2版）

主　　编　刘建平

副 主 编　郑春丽

编　　委　（以姓氏笔画为序）

王　柏　刘建平　何　伟

张文丽　宋文婷　郑春丽

葛　亮　姜　雷

中国健康传媒集团

中国医药科技出版社

内容提要

生物药剂学与药物动力学是药学中的分支学科。本书内容涉及药物的吸收转运、蛋白结合、透皮扩散、代谢消除等动态过程和生物利用度、生物等效性原理和实验方法，以及数据的药动学程序处理等，重点放在基本理论、基础知识和基本技能的理解与掌握。本教材为书网融合教材，即纸质教材有机融合电子教材、教学配套资源（PPT、微课视频等）、题库系统、数字化教学服务（在线教学、在线作业、在线考试），使教学内容更加多样化、立体化、生动化，便教易学。

本教材属于“全国高等医药院校药学类专业第二轮实验双语教材”之一，可供药学类相关专业使用，亦可作为研究生和药剂工作者的参考书。

图书在版编目（CIP）数据

生物药剂学实验与指导 / 刘建平主编．—2 版．—北京 ：中国医药科技出版社，2019.12

全国高等医药院校药学类专业第二轮实验双语教材

ISBN 978 - 7 - 5214 - 1410 - 3

Ⅰ.①生… Ⅱ.①刘… Ⅲ.①生物药剂学 - 实验 - 双语教学 - 医学院校 - 教学参考资料 Ⅳ.①R945 - 33

中国版本图书馆 CIP 数据核字（2020）第 000772 号

美术编辑 陈君杞

版式设计 南博文化

出版 **中国健康传媒集团** | 中国医药科技出版社

地址 北京市海淀区文慧园北路甲 22 号

邮编 100082

电话 发行：010 - 62227427 邮购：010 - 62236938

网址 www. cmstp. com

规格 889 × 1194mm 1/16

印张 5 3/4

字数 124 千字

初版 2007 年 10 月第 1 版

版次 2019 年 12 月第 2 版

印次 2019 年 12 月第 1 次印刷

印刷 三河市万龙印装有限公司

经销 全国各地新华书店

书号 ISBN 978 - 7 - 5214 - 1410 - 3

定价 19.00 元

获取新书信息、投稿、为图书纠错，请扫码联系我们。

序

Preface

教学是学校人才培养的中心环节，实验教学是这一环节的重要组成部分。“全国高等医药院校药学类专业实验双语教材”是中国药科大学坚持药学实践教学改革，突出提高学生动手能力、创新思维，通过承担教育部“世行贷款21世纪初高等教育教学改革项目”等多项教改课题，逐步建设完善的一套与药学各专业学科理论课程紧密结合的高水平双语实验教材。

本轮修订，适逢“全国高等医药院校药学类专业第五轮规划教材”及《中国药典》（2020年版）、新版《国家执业药师资格考试大纲》出版，整套教材的修订强调了与新版理论教材知识的结合，与《中国药典》（2020年版）等新颁布的法典法规结合。为更好地服务于新时期高等院校药学教育与人才培养的需要，在上一版的基础上，进一步体现了各门实验课程自身独立性、系统性和科学性，又充分考虑到各门实验课程之间的联系与衔接，主要突出了以下特点。

1. 适应医药行业对人才的要求，体现行业特色，契合新时期药学人才需求的变化，使修订后的教材符合《中国药典》（2020年版）等国家标准及新版《国家执业药师资格考试大纲》等行业最新要求。

2. 更新完善内容，打造教材精品。在上版教材基础上进一步优化、精炼和充实内容。紧密结合“全国高等医药院校药学类专业第五轮规划教材”，强调与实际需求相结合，进一步提高教材质量。

3. 为适应信息化教学的需要，本轮教材全部打造成为书网融合教材，即纸质教材与数字教材、配套教学资源、题库系统、数字化教学服务有机融合，为读者提供全免费增值服务。

4. 坚持双语体系，强调素质培养教材以实践教学为突破口，采用双语体系编写有利于加快药学教育国际接轨，提高学生的科技英语水平，进一步提升学生整体素质。

“全国高等医药院校药学类专业第二轮实验双语教材”历经15年4次建设，在各个时期广大编者的努力下，在广大使用教材师生的支持下日臻完善。本轮教材的出版，必将对推动新时期我国高等药学教育的发展产生积极而深远的影响。希望广大师生在教学实践中对本套教材提出宝贵意见，以使今后进一步修订完善，共同打造精品教材。

吴晓明

全国高等医药院校药学类专业第五轮规划教材常务编委会主任委员

2019年10月

前言

Preface

《生物药剂学实验与指导》（第2版），是在上版生物药剂学与药物动力学基本理论、基础知识和基本技能的理解和掌握的基础上，根据药学学科的发展要求，听取使用者的意见和建议，对其内容进行充实与更新而进行编写的。通过本轮编写，进一步提高本教材的科学性、新颖性、实用性和可读性。

本教材根据高等医药院校实验教学的新的发展需要，适应生物药剂学的教学要求与学科发展，内容涉及吸收转运、蛋白结合、透皮扩散、代谢消除等动态过程和生物利用度、生物等效性原理和实验方法，以及数据的药动学程序处理等，重点放在基本理论、基础知识和基本技能的理解与掌握。

本书修订工作主要体现在以下几个方面：①补充与更新。根据目前分析技术在药物研究中应用的发展，在家兔体内药动学参数和绝对生物利用度测定实验中增加了高效液相色谱法测定血浆样品方法；根据透皮给药系统研究的深入，在体外经皮渗透实验中增加了体外释放实验部分内容。②调整与改进。根据内容与现行实验课项目改革结合、增加综合性实验的要求，更换在体肠吸收实验药物为磺胺甲基异噁唑（SMZ），与原SMZ表观油水分配系数对小肠吸收的影响实验，共同构建涵盖药物理化性质和动物体内吸收评价的综合性实验。根据实验教学反馈意见，为进一步精准模拟体内过程，对单隔室模型模拟实验的装置进行改进。③纠错与替换。根据对上版教材使用对象的调研，对上版教材中存在错误的公式、符号和缩写进行勘误。对药物动力学实验数据的处理实验中，数学模型原理和回归分析方法介绍不明确部分进行修改。

本教材为书网融合教材，即纸质教材有机融合电子教材、教学配套资源（PPT、微课视频等）、题库系统、数字化教学服务（在线教学、在线作业、在线考试），使教学内容更加多样化、立体化、生动化，便教易学。

参加本书编写的主要人员有：刘建平、郑春丽、王柏、葛亮、张文丽、何伟、姜雷、宋文婷。另外，在本书的内容设计和编写整理中，彭桢、李云、韩涵、邹家辉、王钰、陈名清、李晓彤等同学参与部分工作，在此一并表示感谢。

由于编者编写水平所限，本书中难免存在不足之处，谨请专家、读者批评指正。

编　者

2019年9月

目录

Contents

实验一　磺胺甲基异噁唑（SMZ）大鼠在体小肠吸收

扫码“学一学”

【目的与要求】

1. **掌握**　大鼠在体肠管回流的基本操作和方法。

2. 学习应用在体小肠回流法求算药物的吸收速度常数（k_a）、半衰期（$t_{1/2}$）以及吸收率（单位时间单位面积吸收量）等参数。

【基本概念和实验原理】

小肠是药物胃肠道给药的主要吸收部位。小肠分十二指肠、空肠和回肠，小肠表面有环轮状皱襞和绒毛突起，绒毛上还有许多微绒毛，有效吸收面积很大。由于被动转运速度与表面积成正比，故小肠既是药物被动吸收的主要部位，又是药物主动吸收的特殊部位。

本实验采用动物大鼠在体循环流动法，根据SMZ供试液（含法莫替丁SMZ和酚红）中酚红为大分子络和物，不被小肠吸收，而SMZ可被小肠吸收，同时小肠能吸收或排泄水分子等特点，测定不同时间酚红的浓度，根据浓度变化计算出不同时间供试液的体积，从而计算出SMZ浓度，即可估算不同时间的药物的含量。

【材料与仪器】

1. **材料**　0.2%亚硝酸钠，1%氨基磺酸铵，0.2%二盐酸萘乙二胺（以上置冰箱保存），1mol/L HCl，1mol/L NaOH，生理盐水，Krebs - Ringer 磷酸缓冲液（pH 7.4，每1000ml内含氯化钠7.8g、氯化钾0.35g、氯化钙0.37g、碳酸氢钠1.37g、磷酸二氢钠0.22g、氯化镁0.22g、葡萄糖1.4g），戊巴比妥钠溶液（10mg/ml，大鼠麻醉用，每100g体重腹腔注射0.4ml），SMZ，酚红等。

2. **仪器**　恒流泵、紫外分光光度计、恒温水浴，红外线灯，玻璃插管，离心管（10ml），移液管（50、5、2、1和0.5ml），锥形瓶（100ml），烧杯（500ml），注射器（20ml和1ml），眼科剪刀，眼科镊子，普通中号镊子，小剪刀，手术刀片等。

3. **动物**　大鼠，体重约200g，实验前禁食一夜（自由饮水）。

扫码“看一看”

【实验内容】

一、供试溶液的配制

1. **SMZ溶液（10μg/ml）**　溶媒组成同Krebs - Ringer缓冲液。配置方法为：称取SMZ 10mg和酚红20mg后，加入少量蒸馏水混悬，加入碳酸氢钠并微热使溶解（必要时滴加数滴1mol/L NaOH液）得甲液。另将缓冲液的其它成分用蒸馏水溶解得乙液。将甲液缓缓加入乙液中，添加适量蒸馏水至1000ml即得。

2. **酚红液（20μg/ml）** 溶媒组成同 Krebs－Ringer 缓冲液同。配置方法为：称取酚红 20mg，加少量蒸馏水混悬，加入碳酸氢钠并微热使溶解（必要时滴加数滴 1mol/L NaOH 液）得甲液。另将缓冲液的其他成分用蒸馏水溶解得乙液。将甲液缓缓加入乙液中，并添加适量蒸馏水至 1000ml 即得。

二、大鼠在体肠管回流操作

1. **大鼠麻醉** 将大鼠用戊巴比妥钠溶液（40mg/kg）做腹腔注射麻醉，背位固定于固定台上。

2. **小肠两端插管** 沿腹部正中线切开腹部（约 3cm），在十二指肠上部和回肠下部各插入细玻璃管一支，并用手术线扎紧插入端，另一端分别接橡皮管（图 1－1）。

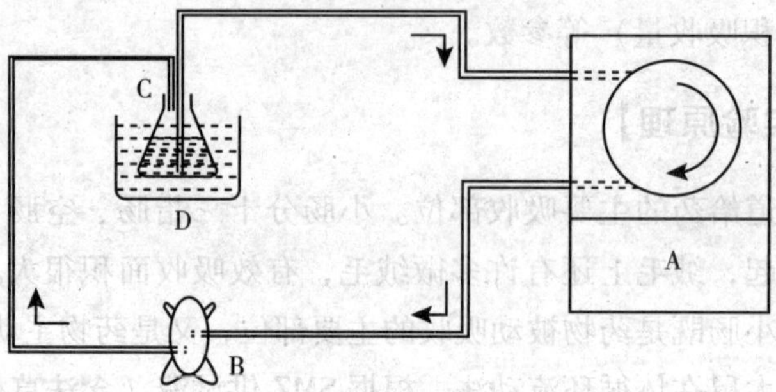

图 1－1 大鼠在体肠管回流装置

A：恒流泵 B：大鼠 C：贮液瓶 D：水浴

3. **洗涤肠管** 将 37℃生理盐水经十二指肠上部玻管缓慢注入肠管，洗去肠管内容物，充分洗涤后送入空气使洗涤液尽量流尽。

4. **肠管回流** 按图 1－1 装置进行肠管回流实验。即吸取 SMZ 溶液 50ml 置贮液瓶中，开动恒流泵进行循环流动，药液从十二指肠上部入肠管，经回肠下部流入贮液瓶中。先以 5ml/min 的流速回流 10 分钟，然后将流速调节为 2.5ml/min，再循环流动 120 分钟。

5. **取样** 回流开始后 10 分钟，从贮液瓶取样两份，一份 1ml，另一份 0.5ml，分别作为药物和酚红的零时间样品。其后每隔 10 分钟亦同样取样两份，每次取样后应立即补充 1.5ml 酚红溶液（20μg/ml）。取样至 120 分钟后停止回流。测定样液中 SMZ 和酚红的浓度。停止回流后，取出回流小肠段冲洗后剖开，平铺于坐标纸上，沿小肠边剪下坐标纸，冲洗后晾干，烘干精密称重。剪取 10 倍（$10cm^2$）坐标纸精密称重后，即求得小肠浆膜总面积（cm^2）。

三、定量方法

1. SMZ 的测定

（1）SMZ 标准曲线 精密称取 SMZ 10mg 溶解在 Krebs－Ringer 缓冲液中，配制成浓度为 20μg/ml 的 SMZ 储备液。吸取该液 0、1、2、3、4 和 5ml 分别加入 200μg 酚红，用 Krebs－Ringer缓冲液稀释至 10ml，得 SMZ 浓度为 0、2、4、6、8、10μg/ml 的标准溶液。分别吸取上述溶液各 1ml，按下述 SMZ 的检测流程操作使显色，在波长 550nm 处测定吸收度，以吸收度－浓度作图，即得 SMZ 标准曲线并计算标准曲线方程。

SMZ 溶液 1.0ml $\xrightarrow{\text{1mol/L HCl 5ml 冰浴摇匀}}$ $\xrightarrow{\text{0.2\% NaNO}_2\text{ 0.5ml 冰浴摇匀}}$ 放置 3 分钟 $\xrightarrow{\text{1\% (NH}_4\text{)}_2\text{SO}_3\text{ 0.5ml 摇匀}}$ 放置 3 分钟 $\xrightarrow{\text{0.2\% 萘乙二胺 0.3ml 摇匀}}$ 放置 20 分钟 ⟶ 在波长 550nm 处测定。

（2）样液中 SMZ 的测定　分别精密吸取样液各 1ml，适当稀释后，按上述方法测定吸收度。根据标准曲线计算样液中 SMZ 浓度。

2. 酚红的测定　精密吸取样液 0.5ml，加入 1mol/L NaOH 5ml 摇匀，用 1mol/L NaOH 作为空白对照液，在 550nm 处测定吸收度。按标准曲线计算酚红的浓度。

四、数据处理

1. SMZ 的标准曲线　将 SMZ 的浓度及相应的吸收度填入表 1-1，并按最小二乘法进行线性回归，得到标准曲线方程。

表 1-1　SMZ 标准溶液的浓度及吸收度

C（mg/ml）	
A	

回归方程：C =

回归系数：r =

线性范围：　～　mg/ml。

2. SMZ 的小肠吸收　计算样液中 SMZ 和酚红的浓度，并填入表 1-2，计算循环液体积和 SMZ 剩余量。

表 1-2　SMZ 小肠吸收试验数据

取样时间（分钟）	酚红 A_p	酚红 C_p（mg/ml）	循环液体积（ml）	SMZ A_s	SMZ C_s（mg/ml）	SMZ 剩余量（X，μg）	lg$X$
循环前	—	$C_{P00}=20$	$V_{00}=50$	—	$C_{S00}=10$	$X_{00}=C_{S00}V_{00}=500$	
$t_0=0$	A_{P0}	C_{P0}	$V_0=\frac{C_{P00}V_{00}}{C_{P0}}=\frac{20\times 50}{C_{P0}}$	A_{S0}	C_{S0}	$X_0=C_{S0}V_0$	
$t_1=10$	A_{P1}	C_{P1}	$V_1=\frac{(C_{P0}V_0+(20-C_{P0})\times 1.5)}{C_{P1}}$	A_{S1}	C_{S1}	$X_1=C_{S0}V_1+1.5C_{S0}$	
$t_2=20$	A_{P2}	C_{P2}	$V_2=\frac{(C_{P1}V_1+(20-C_{P1})\times 1.5)}{C_{P2}}$	A_{S2}	C_{S2}	$X_2=C_{S2}V_2+1.5(C_{S0}+C_{S1})$	
…	…	…	…	…	…	…	…
t_n（n≥1）	A_{Pn}	C_{Pn}	$V_n=\frac{(C_{P(n-1)}V_{(n-}1)+(20-C_{P(n-1)})\times 1.5)}{C_{Pn}}$	A_{Sn}	C_{Sn}	$X_n=C_{Sn}V_n+1.5\sum_{i=0}^{n-1}C_{Si}$	

以 SMZ 剩余量的对数 lg$X$ 对时间 t 作图，得一直线。说明 SMZ 的小肠吸收为一级动力学过程。根据直线斜率求出吸收速度常数（k_a）：

$$k_a = 斜率 \times 2.303 \tag{1-1}$$

根据 k_a 求出吸收半衰期（$t_{1/2}$）：

$$t_{1/2} = 0.693/k_a \tag{1-2}$$

根据下式计算单位时间（h）的吸收率：

$$R_1 = \frac{X_0 - X_{1hr}}{X_0} \times 100\% \text{ 或 } R_1 = \frac{X_0 - X_{2hr}}{2X_0} \times 100\% \tag{1-3}$$

式中，X_0为零时间点 SMZ 剩余量，X_{1hr}为 1 小时时 SMZ 剩余量，X_{2hr}为 2 小时时 SMZ 剩余量。

最后根据小肠面积，计算单位时间（h）单位面积（cm^2）的吸收速率（R_2）：

$$R_2 = R_1 / A \qquad (1-4)$$

式中，A 为小肠浆膜总表面积。

【实验指导】

一、预习要求

1. **复习** 有关的生理解剖知识。
2. **熟悉** SMZ 及酚红的测定方法和原理；小肠插管操作。
3. **了解** 消化管吸收试验法——大鼠在体小肠循环流动法。

二、操作要点和注意事项

1. 小肠插管时，将十二指肠上部剪一小缺口，插入直径为 7mm 的玻管，回肠下部则插入直径为 5mm 玻管。插管后，将小肠小心放回腹腔，注意维持完整的小肠血液供应。在鼠腹部切口部位覆盖生理盐水纱布，并用红处线灯维持体温在 37℃。

2. 洗肠管时，用 150 ~ 200ml（37℃生理盐水）沿十二指肠插管缓慢注入肠管，冲洗去肠内脏物，冲洗速度要缓慢，以免把小肠胀破。

3. 药液先以 5ml/min 的流速循环流动，10 分钟后，将流速调节为 2.5ml/min，并开始计时作为零时间点，然后再循环流动 120 分钟。

4. 由于小肠存在黏膜皱襞、绒毛及微绒毛等结构，因此很难测定吸收性黏膜的真实表面积。大多数情形下，单位表面积的吸收是根据浆膜表面积求得的。

三、思考题

1. 胃肠道中哪一部位是药物吸收的最佳部位？
2. 解释酚红在本实验中的作用，本法可否用于其他药物的小肠吸收研究？
3. 生理因素对药物吸收有何影响？

扫码“练一练”

参考文献

1. 平其能 . 药剂学实验与指导［M］. 北京：中国医药科技出版社，1994.
2. 梁文权 . 生物药剂学与药物动力学［M］. 北京：人民卫生出版社，2003.
3. 高申，钟延强，等 . 法莫替丁肠吸收研究［J］. 第二军医大学学报 . 2000，21（10）：913 ~ 916.

Experiment 1 Absorption of Sulfamethocazole（SMZ） in Rat Small Intestine

Purposes

1. To master the basic operations and method of in situ intestinal circulation technique.
2. To learn how to calculate the absorption rate constant, the absorption half - life and the av-

erage rate of absorption per unit area per unit time according to the in situ intestinal model.

Introduction

The small intestine is the most important site for drug absorption in the gastrointestinal tract. It includes the duodenum, jejunum, and ileum. The outstanding anatomical feature of the small intestine is the tremendously large epithelial surface area through which drug absorption can take place. The large epithelial surface area results from the existence of folds in the intestinal mucosa, villi and microvilli. The microvilli, together with the villi and folds, provides an immense surface area available for absorption. As the rate of passive transport is proportion to the surface area, so the small intestine is the main site for drug absorption by passive transport (especially the duodenum), also a special site for drug absorption by active transport.

In this experiment, the absorption of SMZ is evaluated using an in situ rat intestinal circulation technique. This technique assesses the quantity of SMZ absorbed based on the disappearance rate of the drug from the intestinal lumen solution. Phenol red is dissolved in the drug solution to indicate any volume change of the lumen solution. This dye is reported to be virtually unabsorbed, and it acts as a marker to detected gain or loss of water by the lumen.

Materials and Instruments

1. Materials

All of the chemicals employed in this experiment are analytical grade unless otherwise specified. 0.2% sodium nitrite, 1% ammonium sulfonate, 0.2% naphthalene ethylenediamine dihydrochloride, 1mol/L hydrochloric acid, 1mol/L sodium hydrate, saline, Krebs - Ringer buffer solution ($NaCl$ 7.8g/L, KCl 0.35g/L, $CaCl_2$ 0.37g/L, $NaHCO_3$ 1.37g/L, NaH_2PO_4 0.22g/L, $MgCl_2$ 0.22g/L, glucose 1.4g/L, pH 7.4), Sodium pentobarbital solution (10mg/L, for the anesthesia of rat, 0.4ml/100g i.p.), SMZ (pharmaceutical grade), Phenol red.

2. Equipments

Peristaltic pump, spectrophotometer model, analytical balance, thermo - stable water bath, infrared lamp, L - shaped glass cannula, centrifuge tube (10ml), pipette (50, 5, 2, 1 and 0.5ml), conical flask (100ml), beaker (500ml), syringe injector (20ml and 1ml), eye scissors, eye forceps, normal medium forceps, small scissors, operating blade.

3. Test animals

Rats weighting about 200g are fasted for 12 hours prior to surgery with free access to drinking water.

Procedures

1. Preparation of Test Solutions

(1) SMZ Solution (10mg/ml, contain 20mg/ml phenol red)

Dissolve 10mg of SMZ, 20mg of phenol red in Krebs - Ringer buffer solution to make 1000ml.

(2) Phenol red solution (20mg/ml)

Dissolve 20mg of phenol red in Krebs - Ringer buffer solution to make 1000ml.

2. Intestinal Absorption Procedure

(1) Anesthetization

The rats are anesthetized prior to surgery with sodium pentobarbital solution (40mg/kg intraperitoneally). The anesthetized rats are clamped in place and body temperature is kept at 37℃ by a lamp.

(2) Surgery

The small intestine is exposed by a midline abdominal incision, and two L – shaped glass cannulas are inserted through small slits at the duodenal and ileal ends, as illustrated in Figure1 – 1. The cannulas are secured by ligation with suture, and the intestine is returned to the abdominal cavity to aid in maintaining its integrity.

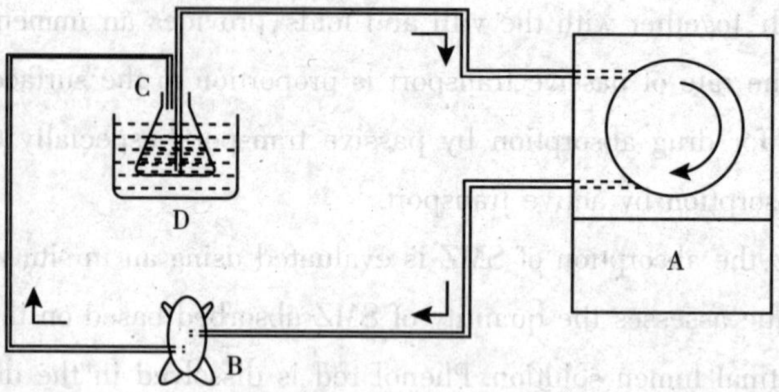

Fig 1 – 1 The device of in situ intestinal circulation in the experiment

A. peristaltic pump B. rat C. liquid storage flask D. water bath

(3) Rinse

The intestine is rinsed free of intestinal contents with saline solution warmed to 37℃.

(4) Circulation

The inflow cannula (duodenal side) is connected by a tube to a peristaltic pump and the outflow cannula (ileal side) to a flask containing 50ml of SMZ solution (Fig. 1 – 1). Then the intestine is perfused at a rate of 5ml/min with the drug solution for a period of 10 minutes and at a rate of 2.5ml/min for another period of 120 minutes.

(5) Sampling

The end of the first perfusion period is considered as zero time point. Sample 1ml for determination of SMZ and 0.5ml for phenol red at the zero time point, after that, 1.5ml of perfusion solution are pipetted separately with a time interval of 10 minutes, and supply 1.5ml of phenol red solution (20mg/ml) immediately. Stop the circulation when sampling for 120 minutes, the concentrations of SMZ and phenol red in each sample solution are determined.

At the end of the experiment, the animal is killed, and the intestine perfused is isolated, opened, spread on a graph paper and dried, then serosal surface area of the intestine is measured.

3. Quantitative determination

(1) Determination of SMZ

Establishing the standard curve of SMZ

A stock solution of 20μg/ml SMZ was prepared by dissolving 10mg SMZ in Krebs – Ringer phosphate buffers. A series of standard solutions (0 ~ 10μg/ml) were prepared by diluting the initial stock solution. 1ml of each solution were taken and the color was displayed according to the following SMZ detection process. The absorbance was measured at the wavelength of 550nm, and plot the absorbance – concentration to obtain the standard curve of SMZ and calculate the standard curve equation.

5ml 1mol/l HCl and 0.2% $NaNO_2$ were added in SMZ solution in ice – bath and standing for three minutes. 0.5ml 1% $(NH_4)_2SO_3$ was added and standing for three minutes. Then 0.2% Naphthalene ethylenediamine was added and standing for twenty minutes.

(2) Determination of Phenol Red

5ml of 0.2mol/L NaOH was added to each 0.5ml of the sample solution. Measure the absorbance of the resulting solution at 550nm.

4. Data processing

(1) The Standard Curve of SMZ

Fill the table (Tab. 1 – 1) for the standard curve and calculate a linear regression equation using the least squares method.

Tab. 1 – 1 Concentration and absorbance of SMZ standard solution

C (mg/ml)	
A	

Regression equation: C =

Regression coefficient: r =

Linear range: ~ mg/ml.

(2) Intestinal Absorption of SMZ

Calculate the concentrations of SMZ and phenol red in each sample solution and fill the data collection table (Tab. 1 – 2) Plot $\lg X$ (X is the remaining amount of SMZ) against time t. A straight line obtained shows that the intestinal absorption of SMZ follows apparent first – order kinetics. Calculate the absorption rate constant (k_a) from the slope of the line multiplied with 2.303, and then calculate the absorption half – life ($t_{1/2}$) by the expression, $t_{1/2} = 0.693/k_a$

Tab. 1 – 2 Data collection table for the absorption of SMZ

Time (minutes)	Phenol Red		The volume of Circulation solution (ml)	SMZ		SMZ remained (X, μg)	lg$X$
	A_n	C_P (mg/ml)		A_s	C_s (mg/ml)		
	—	$C_{P00}=20$	$V_{00}=50$	—	$C_{S00}=10$	$X_{00}=C_{S00}V_{00}=500$	
$t_0=0$	A_{P0}	C_{P0}	$V_0=\frac{C_{P00}V_{00}}{C_{P0}}=\frac{20\times 50}{C_{P0}}$	A_{S0}	C_{S0}	$X_0=C_{S0}V_0$	
$t_1=10$	A_{P1}	C_{P1}	$V_1=\frac{(C_{P0}V_0+(20-C_{P0})\times 1.5)}{C_{P1}}$	A_{S1}	C_{S1}	$X_1=C_{S0}V_1+1.5C_{S0}$	
$t_2=20$	A_{P2}	C_{P2}	$V_2=\frac{(C_{P1}V_1+(20-C_{P1})\times 1.5)}{C_{P2}}$	A_{S2}	C_{S2}	$X_2=C_{S2}V_2+1.5(C_{S0}+C_{S1})$	
…	…	…	…	…	…	…	…
t_n (n≥1)	A_{Pn}	C_{Pn}	$V_n=\frac{(C_{P(n-1)}V_{(n-1)}+(20-C_{P(n-1)})\times 1.5)}{C_{Pn}}$	A_{Sn}	C_{Sn}	$X_n=C_{Sn}V_n+1.5\sum_{i=0}^{n-1}C_{Si}$	

Calculate the average rate of absorption (R_1) per unit time (hour) according to the following equations:

$$R_1=\frac{X_0-X_{1hr}}{X_0}\times 100\%$$

Where: X_0 is the amount of SMZ remained at zero time point, X_{1hr} is the amount of SMZ remained at 1hr time point, X_{2hr} is the amount of SMZ remained at 2hr time point.

Calculate the average rate of absorption per unit area (cm^2) per unit time (hour) by the expression, $R_2 = R_1/A$, where A is serosal surface area of the intestine.

Experiment Guidelines

Requirements for review

1. To be familiar with the operation for the cannula of small intestinal.
2. To be familiar with the principles for the determination of SMZ and phenol red.
3. To know the investigation method for the drug absorption in digestive tract – situ intestinal circulation technique in rats.

Precautions

1. Cut a small incision at the superior part of duodenum and insert a glass cannula with a diameter of 5mm into the inferior part of ileum. Care should be taken to handle the small intestine gently and to reduze surgery to a minimum in order to maintain an intact blood supply. Cover a piece of gauze immersed by saline on the incision. Body temperature of rats should be kept at 37℃ by a lamp during and after surgery.
2. The intestine should be very slowly rinsed from duodenal side to ileal side with 150 – 200ml of saline solution warmed to 37℃.
3. The intestine is firstly perfused at a rate of 5ml/min with the drug solution for a period of 10 minutes, and then at a rate of 2.5ml/min for another period of 120 minutes. The end of the first 10 minutes period is considered as zero time point.
4. Because of the existence of fold, villi and microvilli in small intestinal, the actual surface area of the absorptive mucosa is difficult to measure. In almost all cases, absorption normalized to surface area refers only to serosal (the non – absorptive side), and not mucosal surface area.

Questions

1. What area of the gastrointestinal tract is most favorable for the absorption of drugs?
2. Explain the function of phenol red in this experiment. Whether or not can this model be used to investigate the small intestinal absorption of other drugs?
3. Comment on how physiological factors affect drug absorption.

References

1. Ping Qineng. Experiments and Guidances for Pharmaceutics [M]. The Medicines Scinece and Technology Press of China, 1994.

2. Liang Wenquan. Biopharmaceutics and Pharmacokinetics [M]. People's Medical Publishing House, 2003.

3. Gao Shen, Zhong Yanqiang, et al. Study on Absorption of Famotidine [M]. Academic Journal of Second Military Medical University. 2000, 21 (10): 913 –916.

实验二　磺胺甲基异噁唑（SMZ）表观油水分配系数对大鼠小肠吸收的影响

扫码“学一学”

【目的与要求】

1. **掌握**　表观油水分配系数测定的基本原理和方法。
2. **熟悉**　大鼠离体翻转肠囊法的基本操作和方法。
3. **了解**　药物表观油水分配系数对吸收的影响情况。

【基本概念和实验原理】

小肠有巨大的上皮表面积，是药物吸收的主要部位（尤其是十二指肠）。药物胃肠道内吸收与药物的理化性质密切相关，这些性质包括：药物的脂溶性、溶出速度、解离度等。构成消化道上皮细胞膜为类脂膜，通常脂溶性较大的药物容易通过，而脂溶性较小的药物不易透过，难以吸收。

对于弱酸弱碱药物而言，不同 pH 条件下，药物的油水分配系数不同。SMZ 为弱酸性药物，在 pH 为 4 时吸收最好，pH 增大时吸收速率降低。本实验采用大鼠离体翻转肠囊法，考察不同 pH 条件下 SMZ 的表观油水分配系数对肠吸收速率的影响。

【材料与仪器】

1. **材料**　0.2% 亚硝酸钠、1% 氨基磺酸铵、0.2% 二盐酸萘乙二胺（以上置冰箱保存）、1mol/L 盐酸、Krebs - Ringer 缓冲液（pH 4.5、pH 6.0、pH 7.4）、戊巴比妥钠溶液（10mg/ml）、SMZ 等。
2. **仪器**　恒流泵、752 型分光光度计、分析天平、恒温水浴、氧气瓶、表面皿、试管、注射器、眼科剪刀、眼科镊子、普通中号镊子、小剪刀、手术刀片等。
3. **动物**　大鼠，体重约 200g，实验前禁食一夜（自由饮水）。

【实验内容】

扫码“看一看”

一、供试溶液的配制

SMZ 溶液（10μg/ml）：精密称取 SMZ 10mg 三份，分别加入 pH 4.5、pH 6.0、pH 7.4 的 Krebs - Ringer 缓冲液适量使溶解，并稀释至 1000ml 即得。

二、SMZ 表观油/水分配系数的测定

分别量取上述已配制的三种不同 pH 的 SMZ 供试液 3ml，加入正辛醇 3ml，密塞，剧烈振摇 20 分钟。试验前，正辛醇和缓冲液分别用相应的水相和有机相饱和。离心 5 分钟（3000r/min）后，吸取上层液 1ml，测定 SMZ 浓度，按“四、SMZ 含量测定方法”项计算分配

系数。

三、大鼠离体翻转肠囊实验

1. 大鼠麻醉 取大鼠按40mg /kg的剂量腹腔注射戊巴比妥钠，背位固定于固定台上。

2. 翻转肠囊制备 沿腹部正中线打开腹腔，迅速取出约20 cm空肠段，处死大鼠，在Krebs - Ringer缓冲液（pH 7.4，37℃，通氧）中将肠段冲洗干净，并分为三段，置于含氧饱和Krebs - Ringer缓冲液的表面皿中，用镊子（或玻棒）小心将肠管翻转使黏膜面朝外，分别结扎成5cm长的小囊，每个小囊内加入氧饱和的Krebs - Ringer缓冲液（pH 7.4）0.5ml。

3. 药物测定 将肠囊分别放入5ml pH分别为4.5、6.0、7.4的SMZ供试液试管中，维持37℃和持续通氧条件下1.5小时（如图2 - 1所示），取2ml供试液按"四、SMZ含量测定方法"项测定SMZ含量。

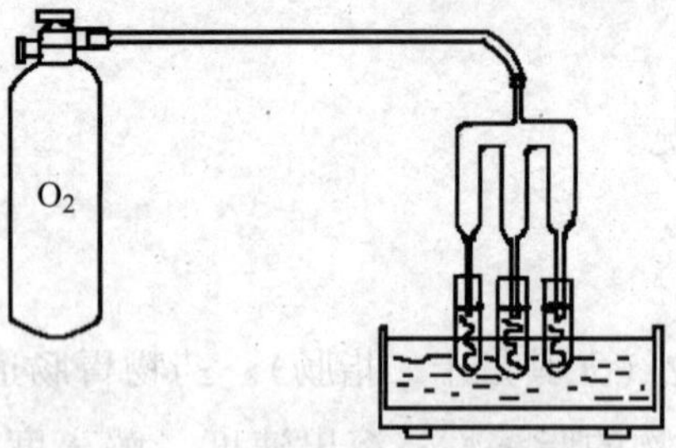

图2 - 1 大鼠离体翻转肠囊实验装置

4. 小肠面积计算 取出肠囊，冲洗后剖开，平铺于坐标纸上，沿肠边缘剪下坐标纸，冲洗后晾干，低温烘干后精密称重。同时剪取10格（$10cm^2$）坐标纸精密称重后，折算成空肠面积（cm^2）。

四、SMZ含量测定方法

1. 标准曲线的制备 精密称取SMZ 10mg，分别溶解在三种pH（4.5、6.0、7.4）Krebs - Ringer缓冲液中，配制成浓度为20μg/ml的SMZ储备液。吸取该液0、1、2、3、4和5ml，稀释至10ml，得SMZ浓度为0、2、4、6、8、10μg/ml的标准溶液。分别吸取上述溶液各1ml，按下述SMZ的检测流程操作使显色，在波长550nm处测定吸收度，以吸收度 - 浓度作图，计算标准曲线方程。

SMZ溶液1.0ml $\xrightarrow{\text{1mol/L HCl 5ml 冰浴摇匀}}$ $\xrightarrow{\text{0.2\% NaNO}_2\text{ 0.5ml 冰浴摇匀}}$ 放置3分钟 $\xrightarrow{\text{1\% (NH}_4)_2\text{SO}_3\text{ 0.5m 摇匀}}$

放置3分钟 $\xrightarrow{\text{0.2\% 萘乙二胺 0.3ml 摇匀}}$ 放置20分钟 ⟶ 在波长550nm处测吸收度。

2. 样液中SMZ的测定 分别精密吸取样液各1ml，按上述方法进行酸化、重氮化、显色等处理，并在波长550nm处测定吸收度。根据标准曲线计算样液中SMZ浓度。

五、数据处理

1. SMZ的标准曲线 将SMZ标准溶液浓度及相应的吸收度填入表2 - 1，并按最小二乘法进行线性回归，求标准曲线。

表2 - 1 不同pH条件下SMZ标准溶液的吸收值

C（μg/ml）	pH 4.5	pH 6.0	pH 7.4
2			
4			
6			
8			
10			

（1）SMZ 标准曲线回归方程（pH 4.5）

回归方程：$C =$

回归系数：$r =$

线性范围：　～　μg/ml。

（2）SMZ 标准曲线回归方程（pH 6.0）

回归方程：$C =$

回归系数：$r =$

线性范围：　～　μg/ml。

（3）SMZ 标准曲线回归方程（pH 7.4）

回归方程：$C =$

回归系数：$r =$

线性范围：　～　μg/ml。

2. SMZ 表观油/水分配系数（$P_{O/W}$）的计算　计算公式为：

$$P_{O/W} = \frac{IC - FC}{FC} \tag{2-1}$$

式中，IC 为最初水溶液中 SMZ 的浓度，FC 为平衡后水层中 SMZ 的浓度。

将三种 pH（4.5、6.0、7.4）条件下的 SMZ 表观油/水分配系数的数据填入表 2－2。

表 2－2　不同 pH 条件下 SMZ 的表观油/水分配系数

pH	4.5	6.0	7.4
$P_{O/W}$			

3. 吸收速率计算　单位时间（h）单位面积（cm^2）的吸收速率 R：

$$R = \frac{X_0 - X_{1.5}}{X_0 \times S \times 1.5} \times 100\% \tag{2-2}$$

式中，X_0 为零时间点 SMZ 药量，$X_{1.5}$ 为 1.5 小时时 SMZ 剩余量，S 为小肠面积。结果填入表 2－3。

表 2－3　不同 pH 条件下 SMZ 的吸收率

pH	4.5	6.0	7.4
R $(h \cdot cm^2)^{-1}$			

4. SMZ 表观油/水分配系数与小肠吸收的关系　将以上所得的数据整理后填入表 2－4。

表 2－4　实验数据处理结果

pH	4.5	6.0	7.4
R $(h \cdot cm^2)^{-1}$			
$P_{O/W}$			

将 R 与 $P_{O/W}$ 进行线性回归，得回归方程，比较相关系数，判断回归效果。

回归方程：$R =$

回归系数：$r =$

【实验指导】

一、预习要求

1. **复习** 胃肠道生理解剖知识。

2. **了解** 大鼠离体翻转肠囊吸收实验的原理；SMZ 含量测定原理。

二、操作要点和注意事项

1. 在翻转肠囊操作过程中，应用镊子（或玻棒）小心将肠管翻转使黏膜面朝外，以防止肠管破裂；另外整个过程应尽可能迅速，以保持离体细胞的活性。

2. 腹腔注射时，左手固定动物，右手持注射器，在下腹部外侧将针头刺入皮下，然后以 45°角刺入腹腔，注入药液。针头与腹腔的角度不宜太小，否则易进入皮下。

3. SMZ 显色反应需置冰浴中进行，反应过程中需要不断振摇并严格控制反应时间。

三、思考题

1. 为什么有些药物制剂需做肠吸收实验？药物小肠吸收实验的目的是什么？

2. 小肠吸收实验有哪些常用方法，各有何优缺点？

3. 油水分配系数对药物的吸收有何影响？

扫码“练一练”

参考文献

1. 陆振达，朱家壁．SMZ 油/水分配系数与小肠吸收的关系［J］．南京药学院学报．1984，15（1）：67－70.

2. 平其能．药剂学实验与指导［M］．北京：中国医药科技出版社，1994.

3. 陈颖，郭建新．翻转小肠囊法研究环孢素 A 口服纳米脂质体在大鼠小肠的吸收行为［J］．中国药科大学学报，2003，34（2），137－140.

Experiment 2 Effects of the Apparent O/W Partition Coefficient of Sulfamethocazole（SMZ）on its Absorption in the Rat Small Intestine

Purposes

1. To master the determination of the apparent O/W partition coefficients.

2. To be familiar with the basic procedures of the everted gut sacs technique.

3. To understand the effects of apparent O/W partition coefficients of drug on its absorption in the rat small intestine.

Introduction

The small intestine is the main site for drug absorption because of its large surface area. The physical and chemical properties of drug are related closely with the drug absorption in gastrointestinal tract. These properties include the lipophilicity, the extent of dissociation, and the dissolution rate of drug. The cellular epithelial membrane is the lipid membrane. This membrane presents the barrier to drug absorption. Usually, the greater the lipophilicity of drug molecule is, more easily drug transported.

For the weakly acidic and basic drugs, their absorptions are affected by environmental pH. SMZ is a weakly acidic drug, whose absorption is found to be maximal at pH 4 and least at pH > 8. This experiment evaluates the absorption of SMZ under different pHs using everted gut sac technique. It is also designed to help understanding effects of the apparent O/W partition coefficient of a drug on the intestinal absorption.

Materials and Instruments

1. Materials

All of the chemicals employed in the experiment are analytical grade unless otherwise specified. 0.2% sodium nitrite solution, 1% ammonium sulfamate solution, 0.2% *N* – (1 – naphthyl) – ethylenediamine dihydrochloride solution, 1mol/L hydrochloric acid, Krebs – Ringer phosphate buffers (pH 4.5, pH 6.0, pH 7.4), 10mg/ml sodium pentobarbital solution, Sulfamethocazole (pharmaceutical grade).

2. Instruments

Peristaltic pump, spectrophotometer model 752, analytical balance, thermo – stable water bath, test tubes, syringe injector, eye scissors, eye forceps, normal medium forecps, small scissors, operating blade.

3. Animals

Rats weighting about 200g are fasted for 12 hours prior to surgery with free access to drinking water.

Procedures

1. Preparation of test solution

SMZ solution (10μg/ml) Dissolve 10mg of SMZ in Krebs – Ringer buffer solutions (pH 4.5, pH 6.0, pH 7.4) in 1000ml flask, respectively.

2. Determination of the apparent O/W partition coefficient of SMZ

3ml of *N* – octanol was added to 3ml of test solutions (mentioned above), respectively. The obtained solutions were hermetically shaked after *N* – octanol and test solutions were saturated with the corresponding aqueous phase and organic phase, respectively. 1ml of the upper solution was withdrawn and determined according to the Procedure 4(2) after 5 minutes centrifugation at 3000 r/min. The apparent O/W partition coefficient of SMZ was then calculated according to the Procedure 4.

3. Everted gut sacs Procedure

(1) Anesthetization

The fasted rat was anesthetized with sodium pentobarbital solution (0.4ml/100g i. p) prior to surgery.

(2) Preparation of the gut sacs

The small intestine is exposed by a midline abdominal incision, and jejunal segment (20cm) was removed rapidly. Then the rat was killed. The jejunal segment was rinsed with Krebs – Ringer buffer solution (pH 7.4, 37℃), and was cut into three sections. The three sections were immersed in the oxygenated buffer solution and everted carefully with forceps (or glass rod). Before both of the ends of 5cm gut sacs were tied, 0.5ml of Krebs – Ringer buffer solution (pH 7.4) were added into the cut gut sacs.

(3) Determination of gut sacs

The everted gut sacs were placed in a sample tube containing 5ml of oxygenated test solution of pHs (4.5, 6.0, 7.4), respectively, under 37℃ (as illustrated in figure 2 – 1). After 1.5 hours the sample solution was taken and determined according to the Procedure 4(2).

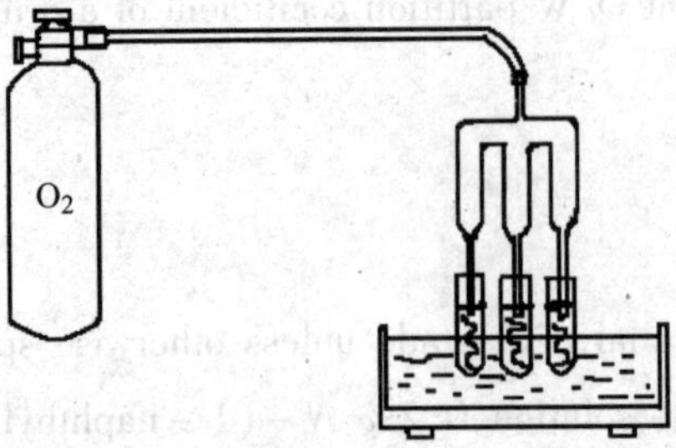

Fig 2 – 1 The experimental deviceof rat gut sacs

(4) Estimation of gut sacs area

At the end of the experiment, the gut sacs were opened and spread on a graph paper and dried in order to measuring apparent serosal surface area of the gut sacs.

4. Quantitative determination of SMZ

(1) Preparation of the standard curve

Stock solution of 20μg/ml SMZ were prepared by dissolving 10mg SMZ in three Krebs – Ringer phosphate buffers (pH 4.5, 6.0, 7.4). A series of standard solutions (0 ~ 10μg/ml) were prepared by diluting the initial stock solution. Measure accurately 1ml of the standard solution, add 5ml of 1mol/L hydrochloric acid solution and shake well, cool with an iced bath, add 0.5ml of 0.2% sodium nitrite solution, shake, cool with an iced bath, let stand for 3 minutes, add 1% ammonium sulfamate solution and gently shake well, let stand for 3 minutes, add 0.3ml of 0.2% *N* – (1 – Naphthyl) – ethylenediamine dihydrochloride solution and shake well, allow to stand for 20 minutes. Calibration curve of absorbance (*A*) versus concentration (*C*, μg/ml) is analyzed by the least – square regression.

(2) Determination of SMZ concentration in the sample

Measure accurately 1ml of the sample solution, and treat the solution as mentioned above. Determine the absorbance of the resulting solution at λ550nm. Calculate the concentration of SMZ in the sample according to the standard curve.

5. Data processing

(1) The Standard Curve of SMZ

Fill the Tab. 2 – 1 with the absorbance and establish the standard curve using the least – square method.

Tab. 2 – 1 Absorbance of the standard solution under different pHs

C (μg/ml)	pH 4.5	pH 6.0	pH 7.4
2			
4			
6			
8			
10			

① The linear regression equation of the standard curve(pH 4.5)

Regression equation: $C =$

Regression coefficient: $r =$

Linear range:　–　μg/ml.

② The linear regression equation of the standard curve(pH 6.0)

Regression equation: $C =$

Regression coefficient: $r =$

Linear range:　–　μg/ml.

③ The linear regression equation of the standard curve(pH 7.4)

Regression equation: $C =$

Regression coefficient: $r =$

Linear range:　–　μg/ml.

(2) The apparent O/W partition coefficient of SMZ under different pHs

Calculate the apparent O/W partition coefficient according to the equation(2 – 1):

$$P_{O/W} = \frac{IC - FC}{FC} \qquad (2-1)$$

where: $P_{O/W}$ is the apparent O/W partition coefficient, IC is the SMZ concentration at the initial aqueous solution, and FC is the SMZ concentration in the aqueous solution after equilibrium.

Fill the Tab. 2 – 2 with the calculated apparent O/W partition coefficients.

Tab. 2 – 2　The apparent O/W partition coefficients under different pHs

pH	4.5	6.0	7.4
$P_{O/W}$			

(3) Calculation of the average rate of intestinal absorption

Calculate the average rate of absorption using the equation(2 – 2) and fill the Tab. 2 – 3:

$$R = \frac{X_0 - X_{1.5}}{X_0 \times S \times 1.5} \times 100\% \qquad (2-2)$$

Where: R is the average rate of absorption per unit area(cm^2) per unit time(hour).

Tab. 2 – 3　The average rate of absorption under different pHs

pH	4.5	6.0	7.4
$R(h \cdot cm^2)^{-1}$			

(4) The relationship between the apparent O/W partition coefficient and the average absorption rate

Fill the Tab. 2 – 4 with above experimental data.

Tab. 2 – 4　R and $P_{O/W}$ under different pHs

pH	4.5	6.0	7.4
$R(h \cdot cm^2)^{-1}$			
$P_{O/W}$			

Calculate a linear regression equation using the least squares method.

Regression equation: $R =$

$r =$

Experimental Guidelines

Requirements for preview

1. To review the chapters concerning dissection of gastrointestinal tract.

2. To learn the principle of the everted gut sacs technique and the determination principle of SMZ.

Precautions

1. During everted gut sacs procedure, the jejunal segment should be everted carefully with forceps against the damage for the jejunal segment.

2. When rat was anesthetized, insert subcutaneously a needle into the inferior belly and then insert it further into abdomen at an angle of 45°. Adjust the angle of syringe needle to avoid injecting the drug subcutaneously.

3. The colorizing reaction of SMZ should be carried out in an ice bath, keep shaking during the reaction and the time should be strictly controlled.

Questions

1. Why are intestinal absorption studies needed for some pharmaceutical preparations? What goal is intestinal absorption studies for some drug?

2. What experimental methods for the study of the drug intestinal absorption are now available and what are their advantages and shortcomings?

3. What is the effect of apparent O/W partition coefficient of drug on the absorption?

References

1. Lu Zhenda, Zhu Jiabi, etc. The Correlation between Small Intestinal Absorbtion of SMZ and O/W Partition Coefficient[J]. Jounal of Nanjing College of Pharmacy. 1984, 15(1):67 – 70.

2. Ping Qineng. Experiments and Guidances for Pharmaceutics[M]. Peking China Medico – pharmaceutical Scinence & Technology Publishing House. 1994.

3. Chen Ying, Guo Jianxin, etc. Everted Gut Sac as a Technique to Study the Absorption Behavi or of Cyclosporin A Nanoliposome[J]. Journal of China Pharmaceutical University. 2003, 34 (2), 137 – 140.

实验三 吲哚拉新两种晶型的制备和溶解性质研究

扫码“学一学”

【目的与要求】

1. **掌握** 测定药物平衡溶解度的方法。
2. **熟悉** 吲哚拉新两种晶型的制备方法。
3. **了解** 药物不同晶型的溶解度差异及其对药物溶出和吸收的影响。

【基本概念和实验原理】

晶型是指结晶物质内分子的排列形式。晶型之间的差异实质上是结晶的基本单元——晶胞微观结构上的差异，这是晶格内部分子依不同方式排列或堆积产生的。同一种物质的分子能够形成多种晶型的现象称为同质多晶现象，许多化合物存在多晶型。

同种药物可能有多种不同晶型，包括稳定型和亚稳型。吲哚拉新是非甾体抗炎药，有4种不同晶型。由于晶格能的差异，不同晶型的理化性质如熔点、溶解度、溶出速度和稳定性等亦不同，从而影响药物的吸收。

药物溶解度的测定方法分为平衡法和动态法两种类型，以前者较为常用。平衡法是将被测药物在恒温下搅拌溶解，达动态平衡后，取样过滤，测定药物浓度即得。

【材料和仪器】

1. **材料** 吲哚拉新，三氯甲烷，无水乙醇，人工肠液。
2. **仪器** 烧杯，培养皿，751分光光度计，吸量管，容量瓶，智能溶出实验仪，分析天平，注射器，微孔滤膜，滤器，取样器，试管等。

【实验内容】

扫码“看一看”

一、α型和δ型吲哚拉新的制备

1. **α型吲哚拉新的制备** 称取吲哚拉新0.12g，置于50ml无水乙醇中，超声溶解，倾入敞口培养皿中，于通风橱内室温挥去溶剂，析出α型晶型。
2. **δ型吲哚拉新的制备** 称取吲哚拉新0.15g，置于25ml三氯甲烷中，超声溶解，倾入敞口培养皿中，于通风橱内室温挥去溶剂，析出δ型晶型。
3. **显微观察** 将所制得的晶体置于载玻片上，在光学显微镜（400倍）下观察结晶形状。

二、吲哚拉新标准曲线的制作

精密称取吲哚拉新12.5mg，置于500ml容量瓶中，以人工肠液定容，分别吸取1、2、3、5、7、8、9ml至25ml容量瓶中，用人工肠液定容，配成系列浓度的溶液，在289nm波长下，以人工肠液为空白对照，测定紫外吸收度，绘制标准曲线，以吸收度对浓度进行线性回归，得回归方程。

三、平衡溶解度的测定

称取 α 型和 δ 型吲哚拉新各 0.3g，分别置于 900ml 人工肠液中，37℃恒温搅拌，搅拌速度为 100r/min，分别于 0.5、1、1.5、2、3、4、5、6、7、8 小时取样 6ml，经微孔滤膜（0.8μm）过滤，在 289nm 下，以人工肠液为空白，测定滤液的紫外吸收度 *A*，按标准曲线方程计算吲哚拉新的浓度。以浓度对时间作图，取渐近线截距计算平衡溶解度。

四、数据处理

计算各样品溶液中吲哚拉新的浓度，填入数据记录表（表 3-1）。

表 3-1　不同时间吲哚拉新浓度测定值

T（小时）	α 型（C_α）	δ 型（C_δ）
0.5		
1		
1.5		
2		
3		
4		
5		
6		
7		
8		

【实验指导】

一、预习要求

了解　晶体的形成过程及影响因素；平衡溶解度的测定原理和方法。

二、操作要点和注意事项

1. 制备晶型的培养皿应洗净烘干，以免影响结晶过程。
2. 应用三氯甲烷时应在通风橱内进行操作。
3. 平衡溶解度的测定需加入过量药物，以保证整个测定过程中有未溶解的药物。
4. 测定平衡溶解度时，可用保鲜膜封住溶出杯口，以防止水分挥发。

三、思考题

1. 何谓药物的多晶型现象？研究药物的多晶型现象有何意义？
2. 测定药物的溶解度有哪些方法？各有什么特点？测定过程中有哪些注意事项？

扫码“练一练”

参考文献

1. 王晶．吲哚拉新多晶型的制备及溶解度的研究［J］．中国药剂学杂志，2005，3（1）：9~12

2. 平其能．药剂学实验与指导［M］．北京：中国医药科技出版社，1994.

Experiment 3　The Preparation and Solubility of the Crystalline Forms of Indolacin

Purposes

1. To master the determination of the equilibrium solubility.

2. To be familiar with the preparation method of indolacin's two crystalline forms.

3. To understand the solubility difference of the crystal forms and its effect on drug dissolution and absorption.

Introduction

The crystalline form refers to the molecular arrangement in the crystalline substance. In fact, the differences between the crystalline forms are caused by the structure difference in the crystal lattice. In other words, the differences are produced by the different lattice arrangement of the inner molecules. The phenomenon that the same molecule of the same substance can form many crystal forms is called polymorphism. Polymorphism is very common in the solid organic compounds.

Therefore, one drug substance may have different crystal forms, but under the specific temperature and pressure, the most stable crystalline form can be called the stable form and all the other forms are the metastable and unstable forms. Because of the different lattice energy, the different crystal forms of the same drug have different physicochemical characters, such as melting point, solubility, dissolution rate and stability, etc. All these are related to the absorption of drugs.

There are two methods for the measurement of solubility, i. e, the equilibrium and the dynamic methods. The former is common in that drug concentration is determined after drug dissolved to equilibrium with stirring the solution under constant temperature.

Materials and Instruments

1. Materials

indolacin, chloroform, ethyl alcohol absolute, phosphate buffer solution (pH 6. 8).

2. Instruments

Beaker, petri dish spectrophotometer model 751, pipet, volumetric flask, dissolution apparatus, analytical balance, injector, microporous filtering membranes, filter, sampler testing tubes.

Procedures

1. The preparation of indolacin α – and δ – forms

(1) The preparation of indolacin α – form

Weigh about 0. 12g indolacin, solve it in 50ml ethanol at room temperature with ultrasonication. Then put it in the petri dish and transfer to the fume to remove the solvent. Ind-olacin α – form results.

(2) The preparation of indolacin δ – form

Weigh about 0. 15g indolacin, solve it in 25ml $CHCl_3$ at room temperature with ultrasonication. and transfer to the petri dish to remove the solvent. Indolacin δ – form results.

(3) Microscopic observation

Put the crystals on the microscope slide, and observe their shapes under microscope(400 ×).

2. Estabilishment of the standard curve

Accurately weigh 12. 5mg indolacin and dissolve in 500ml buffer solution (pH 6. 8). Transfer 1ml, 2ml, 3ml, 5ml, 7ml, 8ml, and 9ml of the solution into 25ml volumetric flasks. Dilute to 25ml with the buffer solution to get the serial solutions with concentrations of 2.862×10^{-6}, 5.724×10^{-6}, 8.586×10^{-6}, 1.431×10^{-5}, 2.003×10^{-5}, 2.290×10^{-5}, 2.576×10^{-5} mol/L. Measure the absorbance of each solution at λ 289nm in UV spectrometer. Then establish the standard curve.

3. Measurement of the equilibrium solubility

Place the excessive indolacin α – and δ – forms (about 0. 3g) in 900ml buffer solution in the intelligent dissolution apparatus, respectively set the stirring speed at 100r/min. Sample 6ml solution at the predetermined intevals of 0. 5, 1, 1. 5, 2, 3, 4, 5, 6, 7, 8 hours. Filter solution by the microporous membrane (0. 8μm). Determine the absorbence at λ 289nm using the buffer solution as a control. Calculate the equilibrium concentration according to the standard curve.

4. Data Processing

Calculate the concentrations of indolacin in each sample solution and fill the data collection table (Tab. 3 – 1).

Tab. 3 – 1 The concentrations of indolacin at intervals

T(hours)	α – form(C_α)	δ – from(C_δ)
0. 5		
1		
1. 5		
2		
3		
4		
5		
6		
7		
8		

Experimental Guidelines

Requirements for review

1. To know the preparation process of the crystalline forms.
2. To learn the measurement method of equilibrium solubility.

Precautions

1. The Petri dish should be washed clearly to avoid the influence on the growth of crystalline forms.

2. It is necessary to conduct the experiment in the hood when preparing δ – form indolacin.

3. It's necessary to use excessive drug in the equilibrium solubility experiment.

4. Use preservative film to envelop the gap to avoid the loss of the water.

Questions

1. What are the drug's polymorphism and the significance for study polymorphism?

2. How to measure the equilibrium solubilities of drugs? To outline the precautions in preparing.

References

1. Wang Jin. The preparation of indolacin's crystalline forms and the research of its solubility [J]. China Pharmaceutical Journal. 2005, 3(1): 9 – 12.

2. Ping Qineng. The experiments and guidelines of pharmaceutics[M]. Peking China Medico – Pharmaceutical Scinence & Technology Publishing House. 1994.

扫码“学一学”

实验四　阿魏酸膜剂的释放实验及体外经皮透过实验

【目的与要求】

1. **掌握**　释放实验与体外经皮透过实验的操作方法；求算 F_D值的方法，并判断影响膜剂中阿魏酸经皮透过总量的因素。

2. **熟悉**　皮肤的构造、药物经皮给药所经历的两个过程。

【基本概念和实验原理】

经皮给药系统是指控制药物通过完整的皮肤进入全身血液系统的新型药物剂型。其具有延长药物作用时间、避免肝脏首过效应或胃肠道降解、降低毒副作用、减少用药次数、改善患者用药顺应性等优点。

药物由经皮给药制剂进入体循环共经历两个过程：首先药物从经皮给药制剂基质中释放到皮肤表面（后称释放过程），然后皮肤表面的药物再经由皮肤进入全身血液循环。因此，制剂中药物的经皮透过总量主要受制剂因素和皮肤因素影响。经皮给药制剂中药物经皮透过总量的影响情况表达式为：

$$F_D = M_{透皮} / M_{释放} \quad (4-1)$$

式中，$M_{透皮}$代表某段时间内制剂中药物的累计经皮透过总量，$M_{释放}$代表该段时间内药物从经皮给药制剂基质到皮肤表面的累计释放量。当 $F_D=1$ 时，表示制剂中药物的经皮透过总量只受制剂因素（即释放过程）的影响；当 $F_D<1$ 时，表示制剂中药物的经皮透过总量主要受皮肤因素（即皮肤表面药物经由皮肤进入全身血液循环的过程）的影响。F_D越小，表示皮肤因素对药物经皮透过总量的影响越大。

【材料和仪器】

1. **材料**　阿魏酸膜剂（自制，阿魏酸含量 $2mg/cm^2$），人造皮肤，透析袋（截留分子量为 3500），KH_2PO_4，NaOH，蒸馏水。

2. **仪器**　721 紫外分光光度计，TK－12D 智能透皮扩散仪，扩散池（包括供给室和接收室），TGL－16C 离心机，搅拌子，试管（10ml），注射器（5ml），移液管。

扫码“看一看”

【实验内容】

1. **阿魏酸标准曲线的制备**　精密称取阿魏酸对照品 0.01g，置 100ml 容量瓶中用乙醇定容，精密吸取 0.05、0.1、0.2、0.4、0.8、1.0、1.2ml 分别置于 10ml 容量瓶中，加乙醇至刻度，定容，于 320nm 波长处测紫外吸光度（A）。

2. **透析袋和人造皮肤的处理**　根据扩散池的大小，将透析袋和人造皮肤剪成适当大小。

3. **pH 7.4 PBS 缓冲液的配制**　精密称取 KH_2PO_4 2.72g 和 NaOH 0.63g，加 400ml 蒸馏水，搅拌溶解即可。配制缓冲液的实际量可根据需要折算。

4. 体外经皮透过实验　向透皮扩散仪中注入适量水，设置温度为（32±0.2）℃，转速为300r/min，扩散池接收室中放入搅拌子。将阿魏酸膜剂贴于处理好的人造皮肤之上，人造皮肤一侧朝向接受室，固定在透皮扩散仪的供给室和接收室之间（图4-1）。向接收室中加入7ml PBS缓冲液，开始磁力搅拌计时，分别于0.5，1，2，3，4，5小时取样5ml，并立即补充5ml PBS缓冲液。同时取一份不含阿魏酸的膜剂作为空白对照，以校正人造皮肤中成分对测定的影响。操作同上，经12000r/min离心5分钟，取上清液在320nm波长处测定各点的吸光度A。

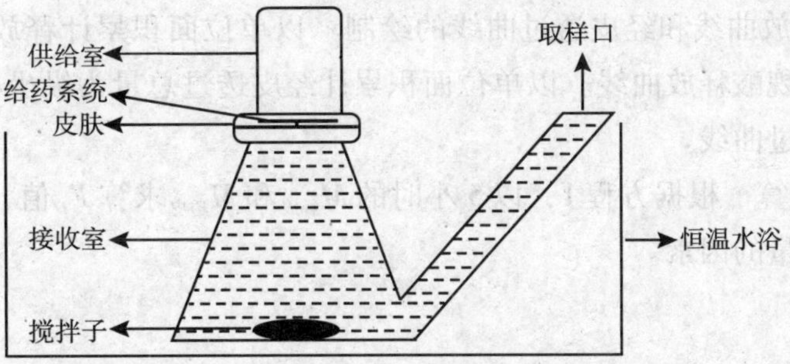

图4-1　体外经皮透过实验装置

5. 释放实验　将人造皮肤换成透析袋，其他操作同“体外经皮透过实验”。

6. 数据处理与实验结果

（1）阿魏酸的标准曲线　将阿魏酸对照品溶液的浓度（C）及相应的吸光度（A）填入表4-1，并按最小二乘法进行线性回归，得标准曲线方程。

表4-1　阿魏酸标准溶液的浓度及吸收度

C（μg/ml）	
A	

回归方程：C＝

回归系数：r＝

线性范围：　～　mμg/ml

（2）$M_{释放}$和$M_{透皮}$的计算　按标准曲线方程计算各时间点的阿魏酸浓度，并填入表4-2，按下式计算不同时间点的$M_{释放}$（阿魏酸累计释放量）以及$M_{透皮}$（阿魏酸累计经皮透过总量）：

$$M = (C_n \times V + \sum_{i=1}^{n-1} \mathrm{Ci} \times V_0) / S(M = \mu g/cm^2) \tag{4-2}$$

式中，C_n为第n点测得的药物浓度（μg/ml），C_i为第i个点测得的药物浓度（μg/ml），V是接收室的总体积（ml），V_0是每次取样体积（ml），S是扩散面积（cm^2）。

表4-2　阿魏酸累计释放量及累计经皮透过总量

时间（小时）	累计释放量		累计经皮透过总量	
	$C_{释放}$（μg/ml）	$M_{释放}$（μg/cm²）	$C_{透皮}$（μg/ml）	$M_{透皮}$（μg/cm²）
0.5				
1				
2				

续表

时间（小时）	累计释放量		累计经皮透过总量	
	$C_{释放}$（μg/ml）	$M_{释放}$（μg/cm²）	$C_{透皮}$（μg/ml）	$M_{透皮}$（μg/cm²）
3				
4				
5				

（3）阿魏酸释放曲线和经皮透过曲线的绘制　以单位面积累计释放量为纵坐标，时间为横坐标，绘制阿魏酸释放曲线。以单位面积累计经皮透过总量为纵坐标，时间为横坐标，绘制阿魏酸经皮透过曲线。

（4）F_D值的计算　根据方程1，以5小时的$M_{释放}$和$M_{透皮}$求算F_D值，并判断影响膜剂中阿魏酸经皮透过总量的因素。

【实验指导】

一、预习要求

1. **熟悉**　释放实验和体外经皮透过实验的原理和方法。

2. **了解**　皮肤的构造以及皮肤对药物经皮透过的屏障作用；经皮给药制剂的特点及种类。

二、操作要点和注意事项

1. 将人工皮肤或透析袋固定在透皮扩散仪的供给室和接收室之间时，应先将其拉紧铺平，否则会增大扩散面积。

2. 接收室加入PBS缓冲液后，应将室内空气排尽。磁力搅拌子的转速以能均匀混合液体为宜，转速太快会形成漩涡，减少扩散面积；转速太小时接收室上、下层溶液难以混匀。

三、思考题

扫码“练一练”

1. 与口服给药相比，药物经皮给药有哪些优点？

2. 经皮给药制剂中的药物由皮肤进入体循环经历了哪两个过程？

3. 如何通过F_D值判断影响经皮给药中药物经皮透过总量的因素？

参考文献

1. 刘建平．生物药剂学实验与指导［M］．北京：中国医药科技出版社，2007.

2. Yogeshvar N，Kalia RHG. Modeling transdermal drug release［J］. Adv Drug Deliv Rev. 2001. 48：159－72.

Experiment 4　Release and *In Vitro* Transdermal Permeation of Ferulic Acid Films

Purposes

1. To master the operation of release experiment and*in vitro* transdermal permeation experiment and the calculation of F_D and to determine the factors influencing cumulative transdermal permeation amount of ferulic acid.

2. To be familiar with the structure of skin and two permeation processes of transdermal drug delivery.

Introduction

Transdermal drug delivery systems(TDDS) can be defined as a new pharmaceutical dosage form which can control the permeation of drug through intact skin into systemic circulation. The advantages of TDDS include extending the action time of drugs, bypassing hepatic "first pass effect" and gastrointestinal incompatibility, avoiding side effects due to the optimization of the blood concentration – time profile, reducing frequency of drug administration and improving patient compliance.

There are two processes of drugs from transdermal delivery preparations to systemic circulation: firstly, drugs release from the matrix of transdermal delivery preparations to the surface of skin(later also known as release process); then, the drugs at the surface of skin permeate through skin into systemic circulation. Hence, the total transdermal permeation amount of drugs is likely to be influenced by transdermal delivery preparations and skin. Guy and Hadgraft proposed the following equation in order to determine the factors influencing the total transdermal permeation amount of drugs:

$$F_D = \text{Fractional rate control by device} = M_{\text{permeation}} / M_{\text{release}} \tag{4-1}$$

Where, $M_{\text{permeation}}$ is the total cumulative permeation amount of drugs through skin from transdermal delivery preparations in a period of time, M_{release} is the cumulative release amount of drugs from the matrix of transdermal delivery preparations to the surface of skin in this period of time. When $F_D = 1$, it indicates that the total transdermal permeation amount of drugs is only influenced by the factor of transdermal delivery preparations(release process); when $F_D < 1$, it indicates the total transdermal permeation amount of drugs is mainly influenced by the factor of skin(the process of the drugs at the surface of skin into systemic circulation through skin). A smaller F_D means a larger effect of the factor of skin on the total transdermal permeation amount of drugs.

Materials and Equipments

1. Materials

Ferulic acid films(self – made, containing ferulic acid $2mg/cm^2$), artificial skin, dialysis bag (molecular weight cut – off 3500 Da), KH_2PO_4, NaOH, distilled water.

2. Equipments

UV spectrometer 721, TK – 12D intelligent diffusion instrument, diffusion cell including donor chamber and receptor chamber, TGL – 16C centrifuge, stirrer, tube(10ml), injection syringe(5ml), transfer pipette.

Procedures

1. Establishment of standard curve

Weigh 0. 01g of the ferulic acid standard accurately and transfer to a 100ml volumetric flask. Dissolve and dilute to volume with ethanol. Measure 0. 05ml, 0. 1ml, 0. 2ml, 0. 4ml, 0. 8ml, 1. 0ml and 1. 2ml of the stock solution into 10ml volumetric flask and dilute to mark with ethanol respectively. Determine the absorbance of each solution at λ320nm in UV spectrometer.

2. Pretreatment of dialysis bag and artificial skin

According to the size of the receptor chamber, the dialysis bag and the artificial skin are cut to an appropriate size.

3. Preparation of pH 7. 4 PBS buffer

Stir and dissolve 2. 72g of KH_2PO_4 and 0. 63g of NaOH in 400ml distilled water. The actual volume of PBS buffer could be converted according to actual need.

4. *In vitro* permeation experiment

The receptor chamberis filled with 7ml pH 7. 4 PBS buffer and the temperature is maintained at (32 ±0. 2) ℃ and stirred at 300rpm throughout the experiment. The ferulic acid film is attached to artificial skin, and then clamped between donor chamber and receptor chamber with the side of artificial skin facing receptor chamber(Fig. 4 – 1). 5ml of the receptor medium is extracted with injector at 0. 5, 1, 2, 3, 4, 5 hours respectively after the application, and an equal volume of PBS buffer is immediately filled up in the receptor chamber. The film without any ferulic acid is dealt with the same method as control simultaneity, in order to correct the influence of artificial skin extract. All samples are centrifuged at 12000r/min for 5 minutes, then the supernatant is removed for analysis, which is performed by determining the absorbance at λ320nm.

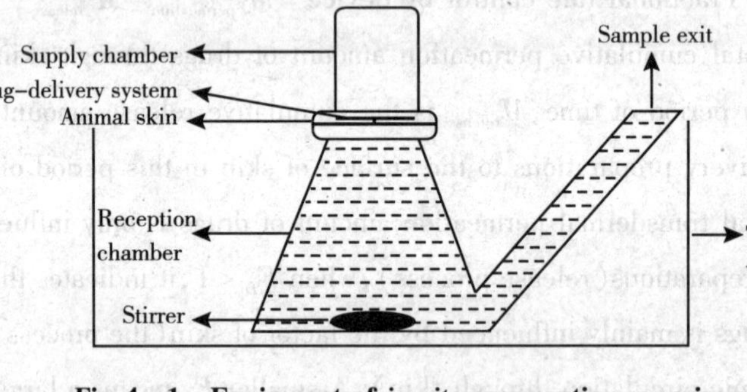

Fig. 4 – 1 Equipment of *in vitro* permeation experiment

5. Release experiment

Except that artificial skin is substituted by dialysis bag, the other procedure is the same with "*In vitro* permeation experiment".

6. Results and data analysis

(1) The standard curve

Fill in Tab. 4 – 1 with the concentration and absorbance of ferulic acid of standard solution. The equation of standard curve can be obtained by the linear regression of concentration of standard ferulic acid versus absorbance of each solution.

Tab. 4 – 1　**The concentration and absorbance of ferulic acid of standard solution**

C(μg/ml)	
A	

Regression equation: C =

Regression coefficient: r =

Linear range:　　~　　mμg/ml

(2) Calculation of $M_{permeation}$ and $M_{release}$

Calculate $M_{permeation}$ and $M_{release}$ according to following equation and fill in Tab. 4 – 2:

$$M = (C_n \times V + \sum_{i=1}^{n-1} Ci \times V_0) / S (M = \mu g/cm^2) \quad (4-2)$$

Where, C_n is the drug concentration of the receiver solution at each sampling time (μg/ml), C_i is the drug concentration of the samples (μg/ml), V is the total volume (ml) of receptor chamber, V_0 is the volume (ml) of sample extracted from the receptor chamber, S is the effective diffusion area (cm^2).

Tab. 4 – 2　**Cumulative release amount and total cumulative permeation amount of ferulic acid**

t(hours)	Cumulativedrug release amount		Total cumulative drug permeation amount	
	$C_{release}$ (μg/ml)	$M_{release}$ (μg/cm^2)	$C_{permeation}$ (μg/ml)	$M_{permeation}$ (μg/cm^2)
0.5				
1				
2				
3				
4				
5				

(3) Release/permeation profile of ferulic acid

The cumulative amount of ferulic acid released/permeated plot as a function of time.

(4) Calculation of F_D

According to Equation 1, F_D is calculated on the basis of $M_{release}$ and $M_{permeation}$ at 5 hours, and then the factors influencing total cumulative transdermal permeation amount of ferulic acid are determined.

Experimental Guidelines

Requirements for review

1. To be familiar with the principles and procedures of release experiment and *in vitro* permeation experiment

2. To know the structure of skin and the barrier effect of skin on drug transdermal permeation.

3. To know the characteristics of TDDS and its categories.

Procedures and precautions

1. Fix artificial skin or dialysis bag tightly between the donor chamber and receptor chamber of

diffusion cell to prevent increasing the effective diffusion area.

2. Make sure that no air bubbles exist in receptor chamber. Keep the stirring rate at a suitable rate to obtain homogenous solution. If the speed is too fast, the vorten will be formed to reduce diffusion area. If the speed is too slow, the upper and lower part of solution cannot be well mixed.

Questions

1. What is the advantages of TDDS comparing to oral preparations?

2. Which are the two processes of drugs from transdermal drug delivery systems to systemic circulation?

3. How to determine the factors influencing the total cumulative transdermal permeation amount of drugs by the value of F_D?

References

1. Jianping Liu. Experiment and guide for biopharmaceutics [M]. Beijing: China Medical Science and Technology Press. 2007.

2. Yogeshvar N, Kalia RHG. Modeling transdermal drug release [J]. Adv Drug Deliv Rev 2001. 48: 159 - 72.

实验五　药物的蛋白结合及竞争作用的研究

扫码“学一学”

【目的与要求】

1. **掌握**　药物蛋白结合测定的透析法。

2. **熟悉**　药物的蛋白结合在药物分布过程中的重要意义。

3. **了解**　水杨酸与华法林的蛋白竞争性结合作用。

【基本概念和实验原理】

药物进入血液后，一部分在血液中呈非结合的游离型状态存在，一部分与血浆蛋白成为结合型药物。药物与血浆蛋白结合后，不能透过血管壁向组织转运，不能由肾小球滤过，也不能经肝代谢。只有药物的游离型分子才能从血液向组织转运，并在作用部位发挥药理作用，然后进行代谢和排泄。

与蛋白质结合的药物和血浆中的全部药物的比例，称血浆蛋白结合率（β）。

$$\beta = \frac{[D_b]}{[D_b] + [D_f]} \tag{5-1}$$

式中，$[D_f]$、$[D_b]$ 分别为游离药物和结合药物的摩尔浓度。

研究药物与蛋白结合的实验方法包括平衡透析、超滤和凝胶过滤等。本实验通过透析过程研究华法林的蛋白结合率。将血浆蛋白与药物的混合液置于透析袋内，使药物与蛋白充分结合后，进行透析。此时游离的药物分子可通过透析袋自由扩散，待扩散达到平衡时，测定药物浓度，即可得到药物的蛋白结合率。本实验还采用该法观测了水杨酸和华法林的蛋白竞争性结合作用。

华法林为抗凝血药物，表观分布容积为0.09～0.24L/kg，血浆蛋白结合率可达99%，属于高结合率、低分布容积的药物，此类药物容易被其他药物（如水杨酸）竞争性置换，与血浆蛋白解离，使血浆中游离药物浓度升高，容易产生不良反应。

【材料和仪器】

扫码“看一看”

1. **材料**　肝素钠注射液，华法林（1mg/ml），水杨酸（10mg/ml），磷酸盐缓冲液（pH 7.4），氢氧化钠溶液（0.01mol/L），乙醇。

2. **仪器**　透析装置（截留分子量为8000～10000的透析袋，100ml烧杯），移液管，试管，容量瓶，磁力搅拌器，紫外－可见分光光度计，离心机。

3. **动物**　大鼠，雄性，体重约200g。

【实验内容】

一、供试溶液的配制

1. 磷酸盐缓冲液（pH 7.4）　精密称取1.36g磷酸二氢钾溶于79ml 0.1mol/L的NaOH

中，加水至200ml即得。

2. 52.9%乙醇　无水乙醇529ml加水稀释至1000ml即得。

3. 华法林溶液（1mg/ml）　精密称取华法林0.1g，加0.01mol/L的NaOH定量溶解至100ml即得。

4. 水杨酸溶液（10mg/ml）　精密称取水杨酸1g，用52.9%乙醇溶液稀释至100ml即得。

二、华法林蛋白结合率的测定

1. 华法林的含量测定

（1）标准曲线的制作　精密称取华法林60mg，加0.01mol/L氢氧化钠溶液100ml，分别量取0.1，0.2，0.3，0.4，0.5，0.6ml药液至试管中，按次序加入0.01mol/L NaOH溶液0.9，0.8，0.7，0.6，0.5，0.4ml，和磷酸盐缓冲液2ml，混合均匀。按紫外－分光光度法，在320nm的波长处测定吸收度。以吸收度对浓度进行线性回归，求得标准曲线方程。

（2）样品中华法林的测定　定时取样测定样品的紫外吸收度，通过标准曲线计算出华法林含量。

2. 透析袋的预处理　将透析管剪成适当长度（10～20cm）的小段，结扎成袋，浸泡于蒸馏水中。

3. 血浆的分离　离心管用肝素处理，大鼠眼底取血约4ml至肝素管中，离心10分钟（3000r/min），分离上层血浆备用。

4. 透析　取血浆2ml和华法林溶液0.5ml于试管中混合，37℃静置1小时后置于透析袋中，将透析袋放置于100ml的烧杯中，内含磷酸盐缓冲液67.5ml，使透析袋内外液体在同一个水平，置磁力搅拌器上搅拌（30r/min），每隔15分钟取透析液2ml，加入0.01mol/L NaOH 1ml，按"二、1. 华法林的含量测定"项下操作，测定华法林的含量（图5－1）。

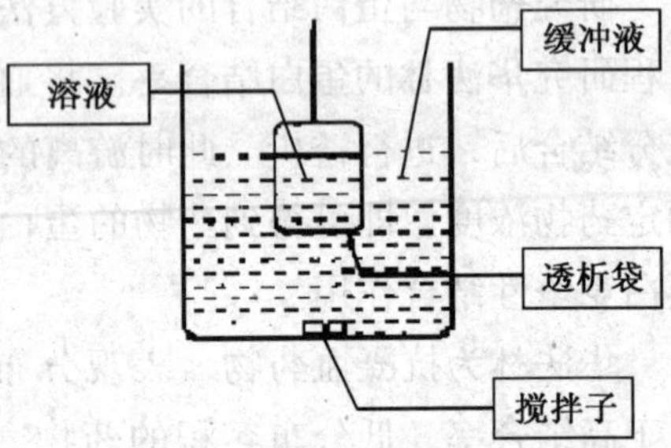

图5－1　透析装置图

5. 蛋白结合率的计算　连续三个时间点的药物浓度相等，说明透析已达到平衡，蛋白结合率按下式计算：

$$E_b = \frac{C_p - C_f}{C_p} \times 100\% \tag{5-2}$$

式中，C_f为透析平衡时游离药物浓度，C_p为药物蛋白混合液平衡时药物总浓度。

6. 数据处理　计算各样品溶液中华法林的浓度，填入数据记录表（表5－1）。

表5－1　华法林的蛋白结合率实验数据

时间 *t*（分钟）	吸光度 *A*	测得浓度 *C*（μg/ml）	透析液实际浓度 *C'*（μg/ml）
15			
30			
45			
60			

续表

时间 t（分钟）	吸光度 A	测得浓度 C（μg/ml）	透析液实际浓度 C'（μg/ml）
75			
90			
105			
120			

表中，C 为测得浓度，C'为透析液实际浓度，$C'=C\times1.5$

三、水杨酸对华法林蛋白结合率的影响

1. 结合率的测定　取血浆 2ml、华法林溶液 0.4ml 和水杨酸 0.1ml 于试管中混合，37℃静置 1 小时后置于透析袋中，将透析袋放置于 100ml 的烧杯中，内含磷酸盐缓冲液 67.5ml，使透析袋内外液体在一个水平面，置磁力搅拌器上搅拌（30r/min），每隔 15 分钟取透析液 2ml，加入 1ml 0.01mol/L NaOH，按“二、1. 华法林的含量测定”项下操作，测定华法林的浓度。待透析达到平衡后，按公式（5－2）计算华法林的蛋白结合率。

2. 数据处理　计算各样品溶液中华法林的浓度，填入数据记录表（表 5－2）。

表 5－2　水杨酸对华法林蛋白结合率的影响

时间 t（分钟）	吸光度 A	测得浓度 C（μg/ml）	透析液实际浓度 C'（μg/ml）
15			
30			
45			
60			
75			
90			
105			
120			

表中，C 为测得浓度，C'为透析液实际浓度，$C'=C\times1.5$

【实验指导】

一、预习要求

1. **熟悉**　水杨酸和华法林的蛋白竞争结合作用原理；透析法的基本操作。
2. **了解**　蛋白结合的概念和意义；蛋白结合率测定的常用方法。

二、操作要点和注意事项

1. 透析袋应提前一天用蒸馏水浸泡，处理时应戴上手套。
2. 透析时应注意控制温度，保持温度在 37℃，透析袋中液面应与缓冲液液面持平。
3. 透析时连续三个时间点测得的药物浓度相同时即说明透析达到平衡。
4. 透析达到平衡的时间因药物不同而异。

扫码"练一练"

三、思考题

1. 简述药物的蛋白结合对于药物分布过程的重要意义。

2. 举例说明药物发生蛋白竞争结合的原理。

参考文献

1. Gonzalez – Esquivel Dinora et al. In vitro characterization of some biopharmaceutical properties of praziquantel [J]. International Journal of Pharmaceutics. 2005, 295: 93 ~ 99.

2. 国家药典委员会编．中国药典（2005 年版）·二部．2005，64，203 ~ 204.

Experiment 5 Drug – protein Binding and Interaction between Drugs

Purposes

1. To master the operation of dialysis.
2. To be familiar the significance of drug – protein binding in drug distribution.
3. To know the interaction of salicylic acid and warfarin.

Introduction

After the drug molecules enter the blood stream, some could bind with protein. Drugs will be unable to reach the tissue after they have been bound with protein, and the drug – protein complex will not be filtrated in the renal glomcrulus. Unbound drug can be freely transported to target organ.

The ratio of protein – bound drug to the total drug molecules is called protein – bound fraction(β).

$$\beta = \frac{[D_b]}{[D_b] + [D_f]} \qquad (5-1)$$

Where D_f is unbound drug, and D_b is bound drug.

The methods studying the drug – protein bindings include dialysis, ultrafiltration, and gel filtration. In this experiment, the fraction of warfarin – protein binding is determined by dialysis. Place simultaneously plasma protein and drug in the dialysis bag to allow them to bind sufficiently. Due to the size of the complex, unbound drug molecule can diffuse out of the dialysis bag. When the equilibrium is achieved, the protein – bound fraction of the drug can be calculated by the determined unbound drug concentration.

Warfarin is an anticoagulant. Its apparent distribution volume is 0.09 ~ 0.24L/kg. The protein – bound fraction of warfarin is 99%. The drug is characterized by the high protein – bound fraction and small volume of distribution. As a result, this drug is prone to be replaced by other drugs (such as salicylic acid) in protein – bound. The abrupt increase of unbound drug concentration in plasma might lead to the serious adverse effects.

Materials and Instruments

1. Materials

Heparin sodium injection, warfarin(1mg/ml), salicylic acid(10mg/ml), phosphate buffer solution(pH 7.4), 0.01mol/L NaOH, ethanol.

2. Instruments

Dialysis bag (cut – off molecule weight is 8000 ~ 10000), beaker (100ml), pipettes, testing tubes, volumetoic flasks, magnetic stirrer, spectrophotometer model, centrifuge.

3. Animals

male rats (about 200g).

Procedures

1. Preparation of test solutions

(1) Phosphate buffer solution (pH 7.4)

weigh 1.36g KH_2PO_3, dissolved with 79ml NaOH solution (0.1mol/L), add distilled water to 200ml.

(2) Alcohol solution

measure 529ml alcohol, and add distilled water to 1000ml.

(3) Warfarin solution

weigh 0.1g warfarin, dissolved with 0.01mol/L NaOH to 100ml.

(4) Salicylic acid solution

weigh 1g salicylic acid, dissolved with alcohol solution to 100ml.

2. Determination of the drug – protein binding fraction of warfarin

(1) Determination of warfarin

① Establishment of standard curve

Dissolve 60mg warfarin in 0.01mol/L NaOH solution and dilute to 100ml. Measure 0.1ml, 0.2ml, 0.3ml, 0.4ml, 0.5ml, 0.6ml of warfarin solution, adjust to 1.0ml with 0.01mol/L NaOH solution, and add 2ml of phosphate buffer solution. Determine absorbance at λ320nm in UV spetrometer. The standard curve is established.

②Determination of the samples

Determine the absorbance of the samples. Calculate their concentrations according to the standard curve

(2) Handling the dialytic bag

Cut the dialysis pipe to suitable length (10 ~ 12cm) segment and form a bag, immerse in distilled water.

(3) Treatment of the plasma

Take blood from the eye of rat, centrifuge it at 3000r/min for 10 minutes, and separate the plasma.

(4) Dialysis

Put the mixture of 2ml plasma and 0.5ml warfarin solution in the testing tube in 37℃ for an hour and transfer it to a dialysis bag. The dialysis is placed in 67.5ml of phosphate buffer (0.064M, pH 7.4, 37℃) in the beaker. Put the beaker on the magnetic stirrer (30r/min). Take 2ml of dialysis solution every 15 minutes, add 1ml of 0.01mol/L NaOH and mix, determine the absorbance (Fig. 5 – 1).

(5) Calculate the drug – protein binding fraction.

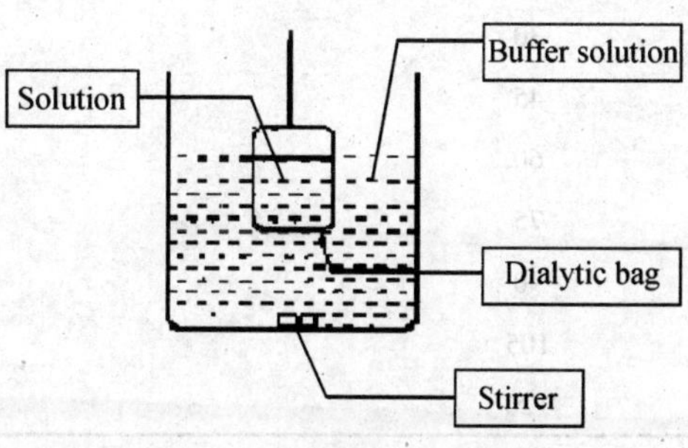

Fig. 5 – 1　dialysis instrument

As the equilibrium of dialysis reaches, calculate the drug – protein binding fraction as follows:

$$E_b = \frac{C_p - C_f}{C_p} \times 100\% \qquad (5-2)$$

Where C_f is the concentration of unbound drug in the buffer solution, and C_p is the total concentration of the drug when the equilibrium is achieved.

(6) Data Processing

Calculate the concentrations of warfarin in each sample solution and fill the data collection table (Tab. 5 – 1).

Tab. 5 – 1 Concentrations of warfarin in the dialysis solution

t(minutes)	Absorbance	*C*(μg/ml)	*C'*(μg/ml)
15			
30			
45			
60			
75			
90			
105			
120			

C: the determined concentration, *C'*: the actual concentration, $C' = C \times 1.5$.

3. The interaction between salicylic acid and warfarin

(1) Determination of the drug – protein binding fraction

Put the mixture of 2ml plasma, 0.4ml warfarin and 0.1ml salicylic acid in the testing tube in 37℃ for 1 hour. Then transfer it to the dialysis bag. The dialysis bag is placed in 67.5ml phosphate buffer (0.064M, pH 7.4, 37℃) in the beaker. Put the beaker on the magnetic stirrer (30r/min). Measure 2ml of dialysis solution every 15 minutes, add 1ml of 0.01mol/L NaOH and mix, determine the absorbance (formula 5 – 2).

(2) Data Processing

Calculate the concentrations of warfarin in each sample solution and fill the data collection table (Tab. 5 – 2).

Tab. 5 – 2 Concentrations of warfarin in the dialysis solution

t(minutes)	Absorbance	*C*(μg/ml)	*C'*(μg/ml)
15			
30			
45			
60			
75			
90			
105			
120			

C: the determined concentration, *C'*: the actual concentration, $C' = C \times 1.5$.

Experimental Guidelines

Requirements for review

1. To understand the mechanism of interaction between warfarin and salicylic acid.

2. To learn the principle of dialysis to study protein binding and interaction of drugs.

3. To learn the common methods of determining the drug – protein bound fraction and the basic procedures of dialysis.

Precautions

1. Immerse the dialysis bag in distilled water before the experiment. And wear gloves to handle dialysis bag.

2. Keep the buffer solution at 37℃, maintain the inner and outer buffer solution of the dialysis at same level.

3. If the measured concentrations of three consecutive samples are the same, the equilibrium reaches.

4. The time of the binding to reach equilibrium depends on the drug.

Questions

1. Discuss simply the significance of drug – protein binding in drug distribution.

2. Give some examples of drugs which interact due to protein binding *in vivo*.

References

1. Gonzalez – Esquivel Dinora et al. In vitro characterization of some biopharmaceutical properties of praziquantel[J]. International Journal of Pharmaceutics. 2005, 295: 93 – 99.

2. China Pharmacopeia. 2nd. 2005. 64, 203 – 204.

扫码"学一学"

实验六　美托洛尔（METO）的体外代谢与抑制

【目的要求】

1. **掌握**　利用肝微粒体进行药物体外代谢及估算代谢参数 V_{max} 和 K_m 的方法。

2. **了解**　大鼠肝微粒体的制备方法。

3. 理解药物代谢的概念和意义；药物代谢抑制的概念和作用；代谢抑制剂对药物代谢参数 V_{max} 和 K_m 的影响。

【基本概念与实验原理】

药物代谢亦称生物转化，是指药物分子在体内经过酶催化作用转变成其他化学结构形式的过程。药物代谢是大多数药物及其他外源性物质主要的体内消除途径。肝脏是最重要的药物代谢器官。根据酶的亚细胞定位，药物代谢酶可分为微粒体酶、胞质溶胶酶和线粒体酶，微粒体酶在大多数药物代谢中起主导作用，而微粒体酶中细胞色素 P450 为人类等哺乳类动物中最为重要的药物代谢酶。细胞色素 P450 又称单加氧酶，由细胞色素 P450 催化的氧化反应基本通式如下：

$$\mathrm{RH(substrate)} + \mathrm{O_2} \xrightarrow[\substack{(2H^+2e^-)\\ \mathrm{NADPH,\ H^+}\ \rightarrow\ \mathrm{NADP^+}\\ \text{NADPH-cytochrome P450 reductase}}]{\text{Cytochrome P450}} \mathrm{ROH(metabolite)} + \mathrm{H_2O} \qquad (6\text{–}1)$$

式中，substrate 为底物；metabolite 为代谢产物；Cytochrome P450 为细胞色素 P450；NADPH – cytochrome P450 reductase 为 NADPH – 细胞色素 P450 还原酶。

药物肝内代谢研究实验方法可分为体外法、在体法和体内法。体外法有多种模型，如 S9、肝微粒体、提纯酶、基因重组酶、肝细胞和肝组织切片，其中肝微粒体适用于细胞色素 P450 参与的代谢研究，亦可用于研究 UDPGT 活性、高通量筛选化合物的代谢稳定性。借助于制备的肝微粒体，加入由氧化型烟酰胺腺嘌呤二核苷酸磷酸（NADP）、葡萄糖 – 6 – 磷酸，葡萄糖 – 6 – 脱氢酶及氯化镁组成的还原型烟酰胺腺嘌呤二核苷酸磷酸（NADPH）产生系统，即可启动药物代谢反应，在体外进行各种与药物代谢有关的研究。

药物代谢属于酶催化反应，可用下式表示酶催化反应的整个过程：

$$E + S \underset{k_{-1}}{\overset{k_1}{\rightleftharpoons}} ES \xrightarrow{k_2} E + P \qquad (6-2)$$

酶催化反应过程分为两步，底物（S）与游离型的酶分子（E）结合形成酶 – 底物复合物（ES），复合物可能重新解离成底物与酶，也可能不可逆地分解成产物（P）和游离型的酶分子；k_1 和 k_{-1} 分别表示结合和解离速度常数，k_2 是形成产物的速度常数。一般可用米氏方程式表示酶催化反应初始速度与反应物浓度之间的关系：

$$\nu = \frac{V_{max}[S]}{K_m + [S]} \qquad (6-3)$$

式中，［S］为反应开始时底物浓度，ν 为反应速度［底物消除速度（$-dS/dt$）或产物形成速度 dP/dt］，V_{max} 为反应的最大速度，K_m 为米氏常数。

（6－3）式两边同时取倒数，可得 Lineweaver－Burk 方程式：

$$\frac{1}{\nu}=\frac{K_m}{V_{max}}\cdot\frac{1}{[S]}+\frac{1}{V_{max}} \qquad (6-4)$$

上式表明，$\frac{1}{\nu}$ 与 $\frac{1}{S}$ 之间具有线性关系，可根据截距和斜率求得 V_{max} 和 K_m；也可直接用初始反应速度与底物浓度，进行米氏方程式嵌合，求得 V_{max} 和 K_m。

药物代谢酶的活性会受到许多因素的影响，有可能发生酶的诱导和抑制。药物代谢抑制可分为可逆性和不可逆性两类；而根据抑制剂的来源，可分为底物抑制和产物抑制；根据对底物代谢参数 V_{max} 和 K_m 的影响，可逆性药物代谢抑制可分为竞争性代谢抑制、非竞争性代谢抑制和反竞争性代谢抑制。前者是指抑制剂和底物结构有一定相似性，与底物共同竞争相同的结合部位，会增加底物代谢的 K_m，但对 V_{max} 无影响；第二种是指抑制剂能和酶的其他部位结合，也能和酶－底物复合物结合，会降低底物代谢的 V_{max}，对 K_m 无影响；后者是指抑制剂仅与酶－底物复合物结合，与游离型的酶不结合，会使底物代谢的 V_{max} 和 K_m 都降低。

本实验借助制备的肝微粒体，加入由 NADP、葡萄糖－6－磷酸、葡萄糖－6－脱氢酶及氯化镁组成的 NADPH 产生系统，即可启动美托洛尔（METO）的代谢反应，并在加入代谢抑制剂的情况下在体外进行与药物代谢抑制有关的研究，包括代谢抑制机理分析。

【仪器和材料】

1. 试剂　美托洛尔酒石酸盐，奎尼丁，NADP，葡萄糖－6－磷酸，葡萄糖－6－脱氢酶，氯化镁，氯化钙，磷酸二氢钾，氢氧化钠，考马斯亮蓝 G－250 染料试剂，牛血清清蛋白（BSA），甲醇（色谱级），高氯酸，三乙醇胺（TEA），磷酸。

2. 仪器　旋涡混合器，冷冻高速离心机，普通离心机，可见光分光光度计，高效液相色谱仪（带荧光检测器），C18 色谱柱（250mm×4.6mm，5μm）。

3. 动物　大鼠，体重 200～300g。

【实验内容】

一、试液的配制

1. 磷酸盐缓冲液（PBS，pH 7.4）　称量 6.8g 磷酸二氢钾和 1.58g 氢氧化钠，置于 1000ml 容量瓶，并用蒸馏水溶解稀释至刻度。

2. 2.0mg/ml 标准蛋白质溶液　精密称量 0.20g 牛血清清蛋白（BSA），置于 100ml 容量瓶，并用 100ml 磷酸盐缓冲液（PBS，pH 7.4）溶解稀释至刻度。

3. 考马斯亮蓝试液　称 100mg 考马斯亮蓝 G－250，溶于 50ml 95% 的乙醇后，再加入 100ml 85% 的磷酸，用水稀释至 1L 即得。

4. 3.75mmol/L 美托洛尔溶液　精密称量 0.2568g 美托洛尔酒石酸盐，置于 100ml 容量瓶，并用磷酸盐缓冲液（PBS，pH 7.4）溶解稀释至刻度。

5. NADPH 产生系统　含 NADP（10mmol/L）、葡萄糖－6－磷酸（100mmol）、葡萄

扫码"看一看"

糖-6-脱氢酶（20IU/ml）及氯化镁（50mmol/L）。

二、大鼠肝微粒体制备

采用 $CaCl_2$ 沉淀法制备大鼠肝微粒体。具体步骤如下：大鼠禁食16小时后，采用断颈处死后剖腹，取冰浴冷却的生理盐水，经胸动脉或门静脉注入肝脏至除去肝中血液，取出肝脏，滤纸吸干水分，称重，并加入4倍于肝重的蔗糖溶液（0.25mol/L），用匀浆器制成匀浆，将肝匀浆置冷冻高速离心机中，于10000g离心15分钟，分离上清液，加入相当于1/10上清液体积的88mmol/L $CaCl_2$ 溶液，置冰浴中放置5分钟并轻摇数次，然后于27000g离心15分钟，弃去上清液，得粉红色沉淀，最后将其悬浮于含20%甘油的0.1mol/L磷酸盐缓冲液（PBS，pH 7.4）中，于-70℃冰箱保存。

三、微粒体蛋白质含量测定

采用考马斯亮蓝法测定微粒体中的蛋白质含量。具体步骤如下：

1. **标准曲线制作**　精密吸取2.0mg/ml标准蛋白质溶液0、0.025、0.125、0.25、0.5、0.75和1.0ml，分别加入去离子水使总体积为1.0ml，加入考马斯亮蓝试液5.0ml，立即旋涡混合。5分钟后以不加蛋白质的样品为空白对照，在595nm测定蛋白质标准溶液吸收值 A。以吸收度值 A 对标准蛋白质浓度作图，进行线性回归得标准曲线。

2. **微粒体蛋白质含量测定**　精密吸取1.0ml待测样品（必要时可稀释），加入5.0ml考马斯亮蓝试液，然后在旋涡混合器上轻微混合，5分钟后以不含蛋白质的样品为空白对照，在595nm测定蛋白质标准溶液吸收值 A，根据标准曲线计算样品的蛋白质含量。

四、美托洛尔含量测定

美托洛尔浓度采用高效液相色谱方法，色谱条件如下：流动相，甲醇-50mmol/L磷酸二氢钾溶液［15∶85，V/V，含1%（V/V）三乙醇胺］并用磷酸调节pH至3，流速为1ml/min；荧光检测器激发和发射波长分别是220nm和295nm；进样体积，20μl。

1. **标准曲线制作**　分别取3.75mmol/L美托洛尔溶液0.67μl、1.33μl、3.33μl、6.67μl、26.67μl及200μl美托洛尔溶液，加入200μl的肝微粒体溶液（2.0mg/ml），加入PBS调节至体积为500μl，混匀后加50μl 60%（V/V）$HClO_4$，涡旋10秒，用普通离心机离心（4000r/min，10分钟），取上清液20μl进样，以峰面积对美托洛尔浓度作线性回归，即得标准曲线。

2. **孵育液中美托洛尔测定**　采用上述“四”中的色谱条件，将“五”和“六”项下孵育液处理后的上清液20μl直接进样，测得峰面积，并根据标准曲线，求得孵育液中美托洛尔浓度。

五、药物体外代谢

取-70℃贮存的大鼠肝微粒体，用磷酸盐缓冲液调节蛋白质浓度至2.0mg/ml；取200μl肝微粒体溶液9份，分别加入3.75mmol/L美托洛尔溶液1.33μl、3.33μl、6.67μl、13.33μl、20μl、26.67μl、66.67μl、133.33μl及200μl，分别加入0.1mol/L PBS（pH 7.4）至体积为450μl，混匀并于37℃预孵育5分钟；然后均加入50μl NADPH产生系统启动反应

（最终体积为500μl），并37℃摇床中孵育20分钟，加50μl $HClO_4$ 终止反应，涡旋10秒后置－4℃冰箱冷却，临用前离心（4000r/min，10分钟），取上清液待进样。

六、药物体外代谢抑制

取－70℃贮存的大鼠肝微粒体，用0.1mol/L磷酸盐缓冲液（pH 7.4）调节蛋白质浓度至2.0mg/ml；取200μl的2.0mg/ml肝微粒体溶液9份，分别加入3.75mmol/L美托洛尔溶液1.33μl、3.33μl、6.67μl、13.33μl、20μl、26.67μl、66.67μl、133.33μl及200μl，再分别加入0.1mol/L磷酸盐缓冲液（pH 7.4），至体积为440μl，混匀并于37℃预孵育5分钟；然后按顺序分别加入10μl奎尼丁（500μmol/L）和50μl NADPH产生系统以启动反应，在37℃水浴摇床中孵育20分钟，加50μl 60%（*V/V*）$HClO_4$ 终止反应，涡旋10秒后置－4℃冰箱冷却。在样品分析之前离心（4000r/min，10分钟），取上清液待进样。

七、数据分析

1. 微粒体蛋白质含量测定的标准曲线　将“三、1”中测得的数据填入表6－1。

表6－1　蛋白质标准溶液的浓度和吸收值

C（μg/ml）	50	250	500	1000	1500	2000
ΔA_{595nm}						

以吸收值对标准蛋白质浓度作图，进行线性回归即得标准曲线。

2. 孵育液中美托洛尔含量测定的标准曲线　将“四、1”中测得的数据填入表6－2。

表6－2　美托洛尔标准溶液的浓度和峰面积值

C（μg/ml）	5	10	25	50	250	1500
峰面积						

以峰面积对美托洛尔浓度作线性回归，即得标准曲线。

3. 药物体外代谢与抑制　将采用“五”“六”项试验方法并采用“四”项“2”方法测得的数据填入表6－3，运用（6－5）式计算肝微粒体液中美托洛尔代谢初始速度。

$$v=\frac{(C_0-C_L)}{C_p}\times V\times\frac{1}{t} \qquad (6-5)$$

式中，C_0 和 C_L 分别为孵育前和孵育终止后测定的孵育液中美托洛尔浓度，C_p 为孵育液中蛋白质浓度（本实验中为0.8mg/ml），V 为孵育液最终体积（本实验中为0.5ml），t 为反应进行时间（本实验中为20分钟）；美托洛尔代谢消失初始速度单位为nmol/min或nmol/min protein。

表6－3　大鼠肝微粒体孵育系统中美托洛尔的体外代谢与抑制

No.	含抑制剂			不含抑制剂		
	C_0（μmol/L）	C_L（μmol/L）	*V*	C_0（μmol/L）	C_L（μmol/L）	*V*
1	10			10		
2	25			25		
3	50			50		

续表

No.	含抑制剂			不含抑制剂		
	C_0（μmol/L）	C_L（μmol/L）	V	C_0（μmol/L）	C_L（μmol/L）	V
4	100			100		
5	150			150		
6	200			200		
7	500			500		
8	1000			1000		
9	1500			1500		

4. 肝微粒体液中美托洛尔代谢动力学参数 V_{max} 和 K_m 估算　可用下列任一种方法估算美托洛尔代谢参数 V_{max} 和 K_m。

（1）利用求得的美托洛尔代谢初始速度和已知的美托洛尔浓度进行米氏方程式嵌合，求得相应的 V_{max} 和 K_m。

（2）将美托洛尔代谢初始速度和已知的美托洛尔浓度转换成倒数，根据 Lineweaver－Burk 方程式，由截距和斜率计算求得 V_{max} 和 K_m。

将本实验两种试验条件下估算得到的美托洛尔代谢参数 V_{max} 和 K_m 做统计学分析，讨论奎尼丁对美托洛尔代谢抑制的机制。

【实验指导】

一、预习要求

1. **熟悉**　药物代谢的基本概念；药物代谢抑制的概念、作用机理和对药物研究及临床用药的意义；

2. **了解**　细胞色素 P450 的分类命名及与药物代谢相关的重要亚型包括 CYP1A2、2A6、2B6、2C8、2C9、2C19、2D6、2E1 和 3A4；细胞色素 P450 重要亚型的常见酶抑制剂；米氏方程中 V_{max} 和 K_m 的意义及 V_{max} 和 K_m 的估算方法。

3. 学习大鼠肝微粒体的制备方法及常见的蛋白质测定方法。

二、操作要点和注意事项

1. 制备肝匀浆物步骤中，自动物体内取出肝脏后，操作应在冰浴中或低温下进行。

2. 微粒体蛋白质含量测定中采用考马斯亮蓝法，其准确性易受去污剂、Triton X－100、十二烷基硫酸钠（SDS）的影响，加入考马斯亮蓝 G－250 在旋涡混合器上混合时不要太剧烈，以免产生大量气泡而难于消除。

3. 微粒体蛋白质含量测定中，必要时可将样品稀释后再按步骤进行测定。

4. 采用肝微粒体进行体外孵育时，最好按顺序并间隔相等时间（如 1 分钟）加入 NADPH 产生系统，以启动代谢反应。

三、思考题

1. 为精确估算米氏方程中的 V_{max} 和 K_m，对微粒体孵育液中加入的系列药物浓度安排有何要求？

2. P450 催化的酶反应中哪一过程为限速步骤？

3. 细胞色素 P450 亚型 2D6 在肝和肠的重要性如何？

4. 采用 Lineweaver – Burk 方程式估算 V_{max} 和 K_m 有何局限性？

5. 在本实验中奎尼丁如何影响 V_{max} 和 K_m？

6. 如果在本实验中采用肠匀浆物作为代谢系统，应用奎尼丁为抑制剂对美托洛尔代谢有明显影响吗？

扫码“练一练”

参考文献

1. Gibson GG，Skett P. Introduction to Drug Metabolism. 2nd ed［J］. London：Blackie Academic & Professional. 1994，217 – 220.

2. Younggil Kowon. Handbook of Essential Pharmacokinetics，harmacodynamics and Drug Metabolism for Industrial Scientists. Kluwer Academic Publishers［J］. 2001，207 – 228.

3. Mikkelsen S. R. Bioanalytical Chemistry. John Wiley & Sons. inc. Publication. 2004，2 – 38.

4. Hemeryck A. DE Vriendt C. A.，and Belpaire F. M. Metoprolol – Paroxetine Interaction in human Liver Microsomes：Stereoselective Aspects and Prediction of the In Vivo interaction. Drug Metabolism and Disposition［J］. 2001，29：656 – 663.

5. Belpaire F. M.，Wijnant P.，Temmerman A.，Rasmussen B. B.，and Brosen，K. The Oxidative Metabolism of metoprolol in Human Liver Microsomes：Inhibition by the Selective Serotonin Reuptake Inhibitors. European Journal of Clinical Pharmacology［J］. 1998，54：261 – 264.

6. Thomas E. Woolf. Handbook of Drug Metabolism，Marcel Dekker，Inc. 1999，203 – 227.

Experiment 6　*In Vitro* Metabolism and Inhibition of Metoprolol

Purposes

1. Understand how to design and conduct the experiment for in vitro drug metabolism using rat liver microsomes, and how to estimate V_{max} and K_m using Lineweaver – Burk method.

2. Be familiar with the preparation method for the rat liver microsomes.

3. Understand the meaning and roles of drug metabolism, and inhibition of drug metabolism. Understand the effects of the inhibitors on the Michaelis – Menten parameters (V_{max} and K_m) of drug metabolism.

Introduction

Drug metabolism or biotransformation refers to as the enzymatic conversion of a drug to a metabolite (or metabolites) , which can be readily excreted into bile or urine. Biotransformation is the major elimination pathway for most drugs and xenobiotics. Drug metabolism occurs in a number of organs and tissues but the major site of metabolism is the liver, due to abundant sorts and quantity of hepatic drug – metabolizing enzymes and hepatic anatomic location. Subcellular Locations of Metabolizing Enzymes are endoplasmic reticulum (microsomes) , cytosol and mitochondria. Microsomes are the primary location for the metabolizing enzymes. Therefore, microsomal enzymes which are heavily involved in drug metabolism are attributed to cytochrome P450 (abbreviated as CYP450, P450 or CYP). The general stoichiometry that describes the oxidation of xenobiotics (R – H) to their corresponding oxidized metabolites (R – OH) is given by the following equation:

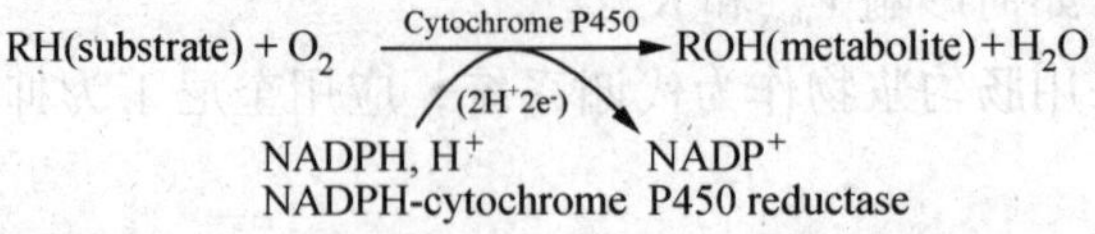

(6–1)

There are various experimental methods for investigating drug metabolism in the liver, including *in vitro* system, in situ system and *in vivo* system. Their application depend on the research objectives. Frequently used *in vitro* system includes S9 fraction, microsomes, purified enzymes, recombinant enzymes, hepatocytes, and liver slices. Microsomes are frequently used because of their advantages in CYP450 metabolism, in the evaluation of UDPGT activity, in high – throughput screening for the compounds of metabolic stability. Various *in vitro* studies relavant to drug metabolism could be conducted in the presence of microsomes following the initiation of the reactions by addition of NADPH – regenerating system consisting of NADP, glucose – 6 – phosphate, glucose – 6 – dehydrogenanse, and $MgCl_2$.

In the simplest case, the overall processes of an initial enzymatic reaction can be described by following scheme:

$$E + S \underset{k_{-1}}{\overset{k_1}{\rightleftharpoons}} ES \xrightarrow{k_2} E + P \qquad (6-2)$$

The enzyme – catalyzed reactions include two stages, i. e., binding of the substrate (S) to free enzyme molecule (E) and forming an enzyme – substrate complex (ES), which then either back to E and S, or further break down to E and product (P). k_1 and k_{-1} are the association and dissociation rate constants, respectively; and k_2 is the rate onstant for the production of P. The Michaelis – Menten equation describes the initil rate of reaction as a function of the substrate concentration:

$$\nu = \frac{V_{max}[S]}{K_m + [S]} \qquad (6-3)$$

Where [S] is the original concentration of the substrate at the beginning of the reaction; ν is the initial rate of reaction or product formation; K_m is the Michaelis – Menten constatnt; and V_{max} is the maximum rate of the reaction.

Taking the reciprocal of both sides of Equation 6 – 3 leads to the Lineweaver – Burk equation:

$$\frac{1}{\nu} = \frac{K_m}{V_{max}} \cdot \frac{1}{[S]} + \frac{1}{V_{max}} \qquad (6-4)$$

The equation (6 – 4) transforms the hyperbola of the Michaelis – Menten plot into a straight line. Thus if the reciprocal of the initial velocity is plotted as a function of the reciprocal to S, we would expect to obtain a linear plot. V_{max} and K_{max} are then derived from the interceptor of the line at the axis representing $\frac{1}{\nu}$ and the slope of the line representing $\frac{1}{[S]}$. Moreover, fitting of the initial velocity versus the original concentration of the substrate at the beginning of the reaction into the Michaelis – Menten equation directly results in the estimation of V_{max} and K_{max}.

The activities of drug – metabolizing enzymes could be affected by a number of factors, and so the inhibition and induction of the enzymes occur. The inhibitions of drug metabolism are divided into the reversible and irreversible ones. Dependent upon the source of the inhibitors, there are substrate – and product – inhibition. Moreover, in the consideration of what occurs to the Michaelis – Menten parameters V_{max} and K_{max}, reversible drug inhibitions are classified as competitive inhibition, noncompetitive inhibition, and uncompetitive inhibition. Competitive inhibition is the simplest form of inhibition, where the substrate (drug) and the inhibitor are very similar in structure and have similar affinities for the same place, i. e. the CYP active site. If it occurs, there will be increases in the K_m of the substrate but no changes to V_{max}. Non – competitive inhibition does not involve the competition of inhibitor and substrate for the same active site. The inhibitor binds to the enzyme at a site distinct from that of the substrate, known as the allosteric site. The expected result is that a decrease in V_{max} is observed without a change in K_m. That is, the affinity of the substrate for the site is unchanged. Uncompetitive inhibition is unusually seen, in which the inhibitor binds only to the enzyme – substrate complex, and not to the free enzyme. Both K_m and V_{max} are decreased in the uncompetitive inhibition.

The animal microsomes prepared in labs could be activated by addition of NADPH – generating system consisting of NADP, glucose – 6 – phosphate, glucose – 6 – dehydrogenanse, and $MgCl_2$. Therefore, inhibition of metoprolol (METO) metabolism including its mechanism could be in vitro studied by the addition of inhibitors to the incubation system.

Materials and Instruments

1. Materials

Chemicals Racemic metoprolol tartrate, quinine, NADP, glucose – 6 – phosphate, glucose – 6 – dehydrogenanse, $MgCl_2$, $CaCl_2$, NaH_2PO_4, Na_2HPO_4, Coomassie Brilliant Blue G – 250, bovine serum albumin (BSA), methanol (chromatographic grade), $HClO_4$, triethylamine, orthophosphoric acid.

2. Instruments

Votex mixer, refrigerated high speed centrifuge, centrifuge Spectrophotometer Model 752, HPLC system (with fluorescent detector), C18 column (250mm × 4.6mm, 5μm).

3. Animals

Rats weighing 200 – 300g.

Procedures

1. Preparation of Test Solution

(1) Phosphate buffer (pH 7.4)

Accurately weigh 6.8g of potassium phosphate and 1.58g of sodium hydroxide, transfer to 1000ml volumeric flask and dissolve in DD H_2O.

(2) 2.0mg/ml BSA solution

Accurately weigh 0.2g of bovine serum albumin, and dissolve in 100ml of the previously prepared phosphate buffer (pH 7.4).

(3) Coomassie Blue G – 250

Dye stock reagent Coomassie Blue G – 250 (100mg) is dissolved in 50ml of methanol. The solution is added to 100ml of 85% H_3PO_4, and diluted to 1L with water.

(4) 3.75mmol/L Metoprolol

Accurately weigh 0.2568g of metoprolol tartrate, transfer to 100ml volumeric flask, and dissolve in 100ml of the previously prepared phosphate buffer (pH 7.4).

(5) NADPH – generation system

A mixture of NADP (10mmol/L), glucose – 6 – phosphate (100mmol), glucose – 6 – dehydrogenase (20IU/ml) and $MgCl_2$ (50mmol/L).

2. Preparation of rat liver microsomes by the method of Calcium Precipitation

Rats are sacrificed by cervical dislocation after 16 hours fasting. Cooled saline solution is infused into the hepatic portal vein in order to remove blood within the liver. The liver is rapidly excised and immediately placed in ice – cold 0.25mol/L sucrose to wash off excess blood and to cool the tissue. The tissue is then blotted dry, weighed and added to four times its weight of 0.25mol/L sucrose. The tissue is finely chopped with scissor and homogenized such that no large pieces of tissue are evident, thereby obtaining a 20% *W/V* homogenate in 0.25mol/L sucrose. In order to obtain the endoplasmic reticulum (microsomal) fraction, the liver homogenate is centrifuged at 10000g for 15 minutes. Aliquots (approximately 10 ~ 12ml) of post – mitochondrial supernatant are mixed with 88mmol/L $CaCl_2$, such that 0.1ml of 88mmol/L $CaCl_2$ is added per ml of supernatant (final $CaCl_2$ concentration is 8mmol/L) and left to stand on ice for 5 minutes with occasional gentle swirling. The mixture is then centrifuged at 27000g for 15 minutes, the supernatant discarded and the pellet resuspended by homogenization in 5ml of 0.1mol/L phosphate buffer (pH 7.4) containing 20% (*V/V*) glycerol, yielding the microsomal suspension. Finally, the suspension is stored at least –70℃ until the protein determination prior to use.

3. Assay of microsomal protein by the Bradford method

(1) Calibration curve for the assay of protein content

By accurately measuring 0ml, 0.025ml, 0.125ml, 0.25ml, 0.5ml 0.75ml and 1.0ml of the previously preparedly 2.0mg/ml BSA solution and bringing all of their volume to 1.0ml using DD H_2O, seven standard solutions (1ml each) containing 0, 50, 250, 500, 1000, 1500, and 2000μg/ml BSA are prepared for the standard assay. The standard solutions are then added with 5.0ml of assay dye reagent and subject to gentle swirling. After 5 minutes, the absorbance at 595nm in the spectrophotometer is measured using glass cuvette and the standard solution without BSA as a blank control. Then, a graph of absorbance at 595nm vs BSA concentration of the standard solutions is plotted. Linear regression could generate a best – fit straight line to the points.

(2) The assay of microsomal protein

1.0ml of the microsomal suspension prepared in Procedure 2 is added 5.0ml of assay dye reagent and subject to gentle swirling on the vortex mixer. After 5min, the absorbance at 595nm in the spectrophotometer is measured using glass cuvette using the solution without BSA as a blank control. Therefore, the protein concentration of a sample could be determined based on its absorbance and the established standard curve.

4. HPLC assay of metoprolol in the incubated solutions

HPLC assay of metoprolol was carried out using a C18 column (250mm × 4.6mm, 5μm) and the mobile phase which consisted of methanol - 50mmol/L KH_2PO_4 (15 : 85, *V/V*), containing 1% triethylamine (adjusted to pH 3 with orthophosphoric acid) was delivered at a rate of 1.0ml/min. The detection was done by fluorescence at excitation and emission wavelengths of 220nm and 295nm, respectively. The volume of injection loaded onto the system is 20μl.

(1) The calibration curve for determination of metoprolol concentration

A calibration curve ranging from 5 to 1500μmol/L metoprolol was constructed by spiking microsomes without the NADPH - generating system being added. That is, 200μl of 6 aliquots of the diluted microsomal suspension (2.0mg/ml) were added 0.67μl, 1.33μl, 3.33μl, 6.67μl, 26.67μl and 200μl of 3.75mmol/L metoprolol in 0.1mmol/L PBS, respectively, and adjusted to a final volume of 500μl (in which metoprolol final concentrations were 5μmol/L, 10μmol/L, 25μmol/L, 50μmol/L, 250μmol/L and 1500 μmol/L). After added 50μl 60% (*V/V*) $HClO_4$, mixed for 4 seconds, and centrifuged at 4000r/min for 10 minutes, 20μl of the supernatant were injected onto the HPLC system. Linearity of the calibration curve was assessed over the concentration range against the responses (peak areas) using least - square regression analysis.

(2) Determination of metoprolol concentration in the incubates

According to the previous conditions (Procedure 4), 20μl of the supernatant of the microsomal incubation matrix obtained from the Procedures 5 and 6 were directly injected onto the HPLC. The integrated peak areas of metoprolol in the elutes was used to calculate its concentration in the matrix according to the calibration curve developed under the Procedure 4 (1).

5. In vitro metabolism of metoprolol using microsome matrix

The stock microsomal suspension was adjusted to 2.0mg/ml protein by addition of PBS (pH 7.4). 9 aliquots of the adjusted microsomal suspension were added 1.33μl, 3.33μl, 6.67μl, 13.33μl, 20μl, 26.67μl, 66.67μl, 133.33μl and 200μl of metoprolol (3.75mmol/L, dissolved in 0.1mol/L PBS), and adjusted to a volume of 450μl with 0.1mol/L PBS. After the resultant matrix was mixed thoroughly and preincubated at 37℃ for 5 minutes, the reaction was initiated by the addition of 50μl of NADPH - generating system [NADP (10mmol/L), glucose - 6 - phosphate (100mmol/L), glucose - 6 - dehydrogenase (20U/ml) and $MgCl_2$ (50mmol/L)] to a final incubation volume of 500μl. Incubations were performed at 37℃ in a shaking bath for 20 minutes; the reaction was terminated by adding 50μl 60% (*V/V*) $HClO_4$. The samples were vortexed for 10 seconds, stored in -4℃ refrigerator. After centrifugation at 4000r/min for 10 minutes, 20μl of the supernatant were injected onto HPLC.

6. Inhibition of in vitro metabolism of metoprolol using microsome matrix

The -70℃ stored microsomal suspension was adjusted to 2.0mg/ml protein by addition of PBS (pH 7.4). 200μl of 9 aliquots of the diluted microsomal suspension were added 1.33μl, 3.33μl, 6.67μl, 13.33μl, 20μl, 26.67μl, 66.67μl, 133.33μl 及 200μl of metoprolol (3.75mmol/L, dissolved in 0.1mol/L PBS), and adjusted to a volume of 440μl with 0.1mol/L PBS. After the resultant matrix was mixed thoroughly, preincubated at 37℃ for 5 minutes, and then added 10μl of quinine (500μmol/L), the reaction was initiated by the addition of 50μl of NADPH - generating system [NADP (10mmol/L), glucose - 6 - phosphate (100mmol/L), glucose - 6 - dehydrogenase (20U/ml) and $MgCl_2$ (50mmol/L)] to a final incubation volume of 510μl. Incubations were performed at 37℃ in a shaking bath for 20 minutes; the reaction was terminated by adding 50μl 60% (*V/V*) $HClO_4$. The samples were vortexed for 10 seconds, stored in -4℃ refrigerator. After centrifugation at 4000 r/min for 10 minutes, 20μl of the supernatant were injected onto HPLC.

7. Data processing

(1) The calibration curve for the assay of the microsomal protein

The absorbance readings at A_{595nm} in the Procedure 3 are to be filled in Tab. 6 - 1. A graph of absorbance at λ595nm vs BSA concentration of the standard solutions is plotted to generate the calibration curve.

Tab. 6 - 1 The calibration curve for the assay of the microsomal protein

C (μg/ml)	50	250	500	1000	1500	2000
ΔA_{595nm}						

(2) The calibration curve for the determination of metoprolol concentration in the incubation matrix

The integrated peak areas in the Procedure 4 (1) are to be filled in Tab. 6 - 2. The calibration curve for the assay of metoprolol is developed by using the concentrations against the responses (peak areas) using least - square regression analysis.

Tab. 6 - 2 The calibration curve for the determination of metoprolol concentration in the incubation matrix

Meto level (μg/ml)	5	10	25	50	250	1500
Peak area (A)						

(3) *In vitro* metabolism and inhibition of metoprolol in rat microsome

Under the HPLC method specified in the Procedure 4, the assayed metoprolol concentrations of the rat microsomal matrix in the Procedure 5 and 6 are to be filled in Tab. 6 - 3. The initial metabolism - based disappearance rate of metoprolol in the microsome matrix is calculated using the following equation (6 - 5):

$$v = \frac{(C_0 - C_L) \times V}{C_p} \times \frac{1}{t} \tag{6-5}$$

where C_0 and C_L represent the nominal and measured metoprolol concentrations pre - and post - incubation, respectively. C_p is the final microsomal protein concentration in the incubation matrix (equal to 0.8mg/ml in this incubation). V represents the final volume of the incubation matrix (equal to 0.5ml in this incubation). *t* represents the incubation period (equal to 20 minutes in this incubation). The initial disappearance rate of metoprolol in the microsomal incubation system could be expressed in the unit of *n*mol/min/min protein.

Tab. 6 – 3 *In vitro* metabolism and inhibition of metoprolol in the rat microsomal incubation system

No.	In the absence of the inhibitor			In the presence of the inhibitor		
	C_0 (μmol/L)	C_L (μmol/L)	V	C_0 (μmol/L)	C_L (μmol/L)	V
1	10			10		
2	25			25		
3	50			50		
4	100			100		
5	150			150		
6	200			200		
7	500			500		
8	1000			1000		
9	1500			1500		

(4) Estimation of metabolic kinetic parameters V_{max} and K_m

Either of the following methods could be utilized to estimate the Michaelis – Menten parameter V_{max} and K_m, which are related to the microsomal metabolism of metoprolol in vitro.

① The profile of the calculated initial disappearance rates of metoprolol in the microsome against the nomimal substrate concentrations is directly fitted to the Michaelis – Menten equation (6 – 3). Best – fitted curve would lead to the appropriate estimation of the V_{max} and K_m.

② By transforming the initial disappearance rate and the nomimal substrate concentrations into the reciprocals, a linear plot called the Lineweaver – Burk plot (6 – 4) results. The reciprocal of rate $1/v$ is plotted against the reciprocal of substrate concentration $1/C$, yielding a straight line with a positive slope of K_m/V_{max} and a y intercept of $1/V_{max}$. The parameter K_m is then calculated from the linear regression values of the slopes divided by the y intercept.

Experimental Guidelines

Requirements for review

1. Understand the concept of drug metabolism. Understand the concept of drug metabolism inhibition, the related mechanisms, and potential clinical significances.

2. Be familiar with cytochrome P450 enzyme system, the nomenclature of CYP450 isoforms, and important CYP450 isoforms including CYP1A2, 2A6, 2B6, 2C8, 2C9, 2C19, 2D6, 2E1 and 3A4. Be familiar with the typical inhibitors of important CYP450 isoforms. Understand the meanings of V_{max} and K_m in the Michaelis – Menten equation, and the method for the assessment of V_{max} and K_m values.

3. Be familiar with the preparation method of the hepatic subcellular fractions (microsomes), the assay methods for tissue protein content, and common interferences.

Precautions

1. In the preparation of the liver microsoms, the operation should be conducted in the cool

bath or on ice after the removal of the liver from the rat.

2. The accuracy in the assay of the microsomal protein amount by the Bradford method is subject to the interferences such as detergents, Triton X－100, and SDS. Avoid the rough vortexed after addition of 5ml of Coomassie Blue G－250.

3. In order to obtain the accurate estimates of the microsomal protein in the stock microsomes, the dilution of the samples may be necessary.

4. In performing the in vitro incubation, the addition of the NADPH－regenerating system should be carefully timed in order to precisely control the incubation time.

Questions

1. In order to accurately estimate the V_{max} and K_m values, what are the general requirements for the arrangement of the nominal substrate concentrations in the spiked microsomal matrix?

2. What is the rate－limiting step in P450－catalyzed drug biotransformation?

3. To discuss the significances of CYP450 2D6 in the intestinal and hepatic drug metabolism.

4. What are limitations in the application of Lineweaver－Burk equation for estimating V_{max} and K_m?

5. To discuss the impacts of quinine on the values of V_{max} and K_m of metoprolol metabolism.

6. If the intestinal homogenates instead of the hepatic microsomes are used, does quinine greatly affect metoprolol metabolism?

References

1. Gibson GG, Skett P. Introduction to Drug Metabolism. 2nd ed [J]. London: Blackie Academic & Professional. 1994, 217－220.

2. Younggil Kowon. Handbook of Essential Pharmacokinetics, Pharmacodynamics and Drug Metabolism for Industrial Scientists. Kluwer Academic Publishers, 2001, 207－228.

3. Mikkelsen S. R, Bioanalytical Chemistry, John Wiley & Sons. inc [J]. Publication. 2004, 2－38

4. Hemeryck, A., DE Vriendt, C. A., and Belpaire F. M. Metoprolol－Paroxetine Interaction in human Liver Microsomes: Stereoselective Aspects and Prediction of the In Vivo interaction [J]. Drug Metabolism and Disposition [J]. 2001, 29: 656－663.

5. Belpaire F. M., Wijnant P., Temmerman A., Rasmussen B. B., and Brosen, K. The Oxidative Metabolism of metoprolol in Human Liver Microsomes: Inhibition by the Selective Serotonin Reuptake Inhibitors [J]. European Journal of Clinical Pharmacology [J]. 1998, 54: 261－264.

6. Thomas E. Woolf. Handbook of Drug Metabolism, Marcel Dekker, Inc. 1999, 203－227.

实验七　对乙酰氨基酚家兔体内药动学参数和绝对生物利用度测定

扫码“学一学”

【目的与要求】

1. **掌握**　高效液相色谱法测定对乙酰氨基酚血药浓度的方法。

2. **熟悉**　残数法计算药动学参数的原理和方法；血药浓度法测定对乙酰氨基酚制剂绝对生物利用度的方法。

【基本概念和实验原理】

1. **静脉给药**　若药物在体内的分布符合单室模型特征，且按表观一级动力学从体内消除，则快速静脉注射时，体内药物浓度随时间变化的函数表达式为：

$$C = C_0 e^{-kt} \tag{7-1}$$

将（7-1）式两边取对数，得：

$$\ln C = -kt + \ln C_0 \tag{7-2}$$

式中，C_0为静注后最初的血药浓度，C为t时间的血药浓度。以$\ln C$对t作图，可得一条直线，由直线的斜率和截距可求出表观一级消除速度常数k和消除半衰期$t_{1/2}$。

$$t_{1/2} = 0.693/k \tag{7-3}$$

$$V = \frac{X_0}{C_0} \tag{7-4}$$

血药浓度曲线下面积（AUC）可由梯形法计算：

$$AUC_{(\text{iv})} = \int_0^n C dt + \frac{C_n}{k} \tag{7-5}$$

全身清除率Cl_s可分别由下面两个方程求得：

$$Cl_s = k \times V \tag{7-6}$$

$$Cl_s = \frac{X_{0(\text{iv})}}{AUC_{(\text{iv})}} \tag{7-7}$$

式中，$X_{0(\text{iv})}$为静脉注射的给药剂量，$AUC_{(\text{iv})}$为静脉注射给药血药浓度-时间曲线下面积。

2. **口服给药**　当药物按体内表观一级吸收过程进入体内，又按一级过程消除，且在体内按单室模型分布时，体内药物浓度随时间变化的表达式为：

$$C = \frac{k_a F X_o}{V(k_a - k)}(e^{-kt} - e^{-k_a t}) \tag{7-8}$$

式中，C为任意时间血药浓度，X_o为给药剂量，F为吸收分数，V为表观分布容积。

假设$k_a > k$，若t充分大时，$e^{-k_a t}$将趋于零，则上式简化为：

$$C = \frac{k_a F X_o}{V(k_a - k)} e^{-kt} \tag{7-9}$$

用常用对数表达为：

$$\ln C = -kt + \ln \frac{k_a F X_0}{V(k_a - k)} \tag{7-10}$$

以 $\ln C$ 对 t 作图可得一条直线，由直线的斜率可求出 k 和 $t_{1/2}$。

吸收速度常数 k_a，则可由残数法求算，将式（7－8）移项得：

$$\frac{k_aFX_o}{V(k_a-k)}e^{-kt}-C=\frac{k_aFX_0}{V(k_a-k)}e^{-k_at} \tag{7-11}$$

设

$$\frac{k_aFX_o}{V(k_a-k)}e^{-kt}=C' \tag{7-12}$$

可以得到，

$$C-C'=\frac{k_aFX_o}{V(k_a-k)}e^{-k_at} \tag{7-13}$$

则（7－13）经整理并以对数表示为：

$$\ln(C'-C)=-k_at+\ln\frac{k_aFX_o}{V(k_a-k)} \tag{7-14}$$

将实验中血药浓度对数－时间曲线的尾段直线外推至纵轴，则吸收期中各时间在该直线上相应的浓度为 C'，C 为对应时间的实测血药浓度值，用 $\ln(C'-C)$ 对 t 作图时，可得第二条直线，称为残数线，从该直线的斜率即可求出 k_a 值。

3. 绝对生物利用度 生物利用度是指药物吸收进入人体循环的速度与程度。生物利用度可分绝对生物利用度 F 与相对生利用度 F_r，绝对生物利用度是以静脉注射制剂为参比制剂，通常用于原料药及新剂型的研究，而相对生物利用度则用于评价不同剂型或同种剂型不同制剂，一般以市售的相同或相近的制剂为参比制剂。

$$F=\frac{AUC_{(\mathrm{po})}/Dose_{(\mathrm{po})}}{AUC_{(\mathrm{iv})}/Dose_{(\mathrm{iv})}}\times100\% \tag{7-15}$$

为克服个体差异对实验结果的影响，每个受试者应在不同时期分别服用受试制剂和参比制剂，并采用双周期的交叉实验设计，以抵消实验时间可能对实验结果的影响。

【材料与仪器】

1. 材料 受试制剂 A：对乙酰氨基酚片（市售制剂，每片 300mg）；参比制剂 B：对乙酰氨基酚注射液（市售制剂，100mg/ml），1% 肝素钠溶液，生理盐水，10% 高氯酸溶液，甲醇（色谱纯），重蒸水。

2. 仪器 高效液相色谱仪，旋涡混合器，离心机，注射器（50ml），家兔固定木盒，红外灯，灌胃器，刀片，烧杯等。

3. 动物 家兔，体重约 2.5kg，实验前禁食一夜（自由饮水）。

【实验内容】

扫码“看一看”

一、对乙酰氨基酚标准曲线的制备

1. 标准曲线的制备 精密称取对乙酰氨基酚对照品，以 50% 甲醇－水配制 2000μg/ml 的贮备液。吸取贮备液 0.1，0.2，0.5，1，2，5，10ml 分别至 10ml 容量瓶中，加入 50% 甲醇－水至刻度，摇匀，得对乙酰氨基酚系列工作液。

精密移取上述各工作液 20μl，各加入空白血浆 80μl，得浓度分别为 4μg/ml、8μg/ml、

20μg/ml、40μg/ml、80μg/ml、200μg/ml、400μg/ml 的标准工作液（C），分别加入 100μl 10% 高氯酸溶液，涡旋混匀，离心 10 分钟（12000r/min），取上清液 20μl 进样分析，记录色谱图与峰面积（A）。以峰面积（A）对标准工作液浓度 C 计算标准曲线方程。

2. 色谱条件

色谱柱：ODS C_{18}（150mm×4.6mm，5mm）

流动相：甲醇－水（30：70））

检测波长：272nm

流速：1.0ml/min

柱温：30℃

进样体积：20ml

二、家兔给药取血操作方法

1. 给药设计　取家兔 6 只，称重，随机分成两组，每组 3 只。第一周期：第一组灌胃给予受试制剂 A（对乙酰氨基酚片用 40ml 生理盐水溶解稀释）；第二组静脉给予参比试剂 B（剂量 100mg/kg）。清洗 1 周后，第二周期：第一组静脉给予参比试剂，第二组灌胃给予受试制剂。每次给药前，先由家兔耳缘静脉取空白血 0.5ml，置于涂有肝素的 EP 管中。

2. 血样采集　给药后，于 0.25、0.5、1、1.5、2、3、4、6、8、10、12、24 小时耳缘静脉取血约 0.5ml，置于涂有肝素的 EP 管中，离心 10 分钟（3000r/min），取上层血浆备用。

三、血浆样品的定量方法

取血浆样品 100μl 置于 EP 管中，分别加入 100μl 10% 高氯酸溶液，涡旋混匀，离心 10 分钟（12000r/min），取上清液 20μl 进样分析，记录色谱图与峰面积。

四、数据处理

1. 对乙酰氨基酚血浆样品的标准曲线　将对乙酰氨基酚标准工作液测得的峰面积，填入表 7－1，并按最小二乘法进行线性回归，求出标准曲线。

表 7－1　对乙酰氨基酚标准工作液的峰面积

C（μg/ml）	
峰面积（A）	

回归方程：C =

回归系数：r =

线性范围：　～　μg/ml。

2. 静脉给药数据处理　将静脉给药后取样所测得的样品峰面积（A）和由标准曲线方程计算所得对乙酰氨基酚浓度值数据填入表 7－2。

表 7－2　参比制剂 B 对乙酰氨基酚注射液静脉给药的血药浓度

取样时间（小时）	0.25	0.5	1	1.5	2	3	4	6	8	10	12	24
A												
C												

求算 k、$t_{1/2}$、C_0、V、和 $AUC_{(iv)}$，由两种方法计算 Cl_s。

3. 口服给药数据处理 将口服给药后取样所测得的样品峰面积 A 和由标准曲线方程计算所得对乙酰氨基酚浓度值数据填入表 7－3。

表 7－3 受试制剂 A 对乙酰氨基酚片口服给药的血药浓度

时间(小时)	A	C	$\ln C$	C'	$C'-C$	$\ln(C'-C)$
0.25						
0.5						
1						
1.5						
2						
3						
4						
6						
8						
10						
12						
24						

求算 k，k_a，$t_{1/2}$ 和 $AUC_{(po)}$。

4. 绝对生物利用度 F 按公式（7－15）计算绝对生物利用度 F。

5. 药物动力学参数 将上述各结果填入表 7－4。

表 7－4 静脉注射和口服给药的药动学参数

	k (h^{-1})	$t_{1/2}$ (h)	k_a (h^{-1})	V (ml)	Cl_s (ml/h) (kV)	AUC (h·μg/ml)	Cl_s (ml/h) (X_0/AUC)
静脉注射口服给药			—	—	—		—

6. 总结 将实验结果进行统计处理，求出平均值和标准差，计算各参数，填入表 7－5，根据计算结果，作 $\ln C-t$ 图，将各有关参数按公式（7－1）和（7－8）得静脉及口服给药后血药浓度的经时表达式。

表 7－5 静脉与口服给药的血药浓度及其参数平均值（n＝6）

取样时间(小时)	静脉注射血药浓度兔号							口服给药血药浓度兔号						
	1	2	3	4	5	6	$\bar{x}\pm s$	1	2	3	4	5	6	$\bar{x}\pm s$
0.25														
0.5														
1														
1.5														
2														
3														
4														

续表

取样时间（小时）	静脉注射血药浓度兔号							口服给药血药浓度兔号						
	1	2	3	4	5	6	$\bar{x}\pm s$	1	2	3	4	5	6	$\bar{x}\pm s$
6														
8														
10														
12														
24														
k（h^{-1}）														
AUC（h·μg/ml）														
F（%）														

【实验指导】

一、预习要求

1. **复习**　药理学实验相关操作方法（静脉注射、灌胃给药和耳缘静脉取血）。
2. **复习**　单隔室药动学的基本概念和原理。
3. **熟悉**　高效液相色谱测定的基本操作。
3. **了解**　对乙酰氨基酚血浆浓度的测定原理；数据处理方法。

二、操作要点和注意事项

1. 口服给药时，先将家兔固定，再将开口器置入家兔口上下门牙之间，用弯钳药片小心送入咽喉部，再用适量水将药片冲入胃中。

2. 耳缘静脉注射时先拔去耳缘外侧静脉处毛，用左手拇指和中指捏住耳尖部，食指垫在兔耳注射处的下面。右手持注射器，先从耳尖端开始注射，刺入后用左手拇指、食指及中指捏住针头接头处及兔耳加以固定，以防突然挣扎时针尖脱出血管。

3. 为避免凝血，试管应预先用1%的肝素钠均匀地浸湿试管壁，放入80℃的烘箱中烤干备用。

4. 溶血是由于各种因素造成红细胞破坏，胞内血红蛋白等物质和细胞内液进入血浆的现象，会直接影响检验结果的准确性。为避免溶血，在取血过程中应避免用力挤压取血部位，取血进入试管时应沿试管壁缓慢流入。

三、思考题

1. 简述药动学实验中采用残数法处理数据的条件和步骤。
2. 本实验中介绍了哪两种求算全身清除率的方法？试比较两者的优缺点。

扫码“练一练”

参考文献

1. 张君仁．体内药物分析［M］．北京：化学工业出版社，2002.
2. 梁文权．生物药剂学与药物动力学［M］．北京：人民卫生出版社，2003.

Experiment 7 Estimation of Pharmacokinetic Parameters and Absolute Bioavailability of Acetaminophen in rabbits

Purposes

1. To master the determination method of rabbit blood concentration of acetaminophen.

2. To be familiar with theestimation of pharmacokinetics parameters, and the estimation of the absolute bioavailability.

Introduction

1. Intravenous injection

Following rapid intravenous injection of a drug that distributes in the body according to a one-compartment model and is eliminated by apparent first-order kinetics, the time course ofplasma concentration of drug is given by

$$C = C_0 e^{-kt} \tag{7-1}$$

Taking the common logarithm of both sides of Eq. (7-1) gives

$$\ln C = -kt + \ln C_0 \tag{7-2}$$

where C_0 is the drug concentration in plasma immediately after injection. C is the drug concentration in the plasma at time$t$after injection. Eq. (7-4) indicates that a plot of $\ln C$ versus t will be linear under the conditions stated. Hence the elimination rate constant and the elimination half life may be estimated from plots of log drug concentration in plasma versus time.

$$t_{1/2} = 0.693/k \tag{7-3}$$

$$V = \frac{X_0}{C_0} \tag{7-4}$$

C_0 may be obtained by extrapolation of the log C versus t plot to time zero. This intercept, C_0, may be used in the calculation of the apparent volume of distribution.

The total area under the plasma drug concentration-time curve AUC is calculated using the trapezoidal rule.

$$AUC\text{iv} = \int_0^n C dt + \frac{C_n}{k} \tag{7-5}$$

Systemic clearance Cl_s can be calculated using two following Eq. (7-6) and (7-7):

$$Cl_s = k \times V \tag{7-6}$$

$$Cl_s = \frac{X_{0(\text{iv})}}{AUC_{(\text{iv})}} \tag{7-7}$$

where $X_{0(\text{iv})}$ is the intravenous dose and $AUC_{(\text{iv})}$ is the total area under the plasma drug concentration-time curve intravenously.

2. Oral administration

When drug performs first-order absorption, first-order elimination and one compartment model distribution, the time course of plasma concentration of drug is given by

$$C = \frac{k_a F X_o}{V(k_a - k)}(e^{-kt} - e^{-k_a t}) \tag{7-8}$$

where C is blood drug concentration at any time, X_0 is administration dosage, F is absorption fraction, V is apparent volume of distribution.

For most of drugs, $k_a > k$, then e^{-kat} tends to be zero when t is long enough, Eq. (7－8) can be simplified:

$$C = \frac{k_a F X_o}{V(k_a - k)} e^{-kt} \tag{7-9}$$

Rewrite it using common logarithm then we get (7－10):

$$\ln C = -kt + \ln \frac{k_a F X_0}{V(k_a - k)} \tag{7-10}$$

In this formulation, a line is established at the post－phase of the curve of log blood drug concentration versus time, then elimination rate constant k and elimination half life $t_{1/2}$ can be calculated from the slope rate of this line.

Absorption rate constant k_a can be calculated by residual method. Eq. (7－8) can be rewritten to Eq. (7－11):

$$\frac{k_a F X_o}{V(k_a - k)} e^{-kt} \quad C = \frac{k_a F X_0}{V(k_a - k)} e^{-k_a t} \tag{7-11}$$

Then let

$$\frac{k_a F X_o}{V(k_a - k)} e^{-kt} = C' \tag{7-12}$$

We get the equation below:

$$C - C' = \frac{k_a F X_o}{V(k_a - k)} e^{-k_a t} \tag{7-13}$$

Calculate Eq. (7－13) using log at both sides, then:

$$\ln(C' - C) = -k_a t + \ln \frac{k_a F X_o}{V(k_a - k)} \tag{7-14}$$

We can get C', drug concentration at the period of absorption, by linear extrapolation of the curve of blood drug concentration versus time to Y－axis. Plot $\ln(C' - C)$ versus time t, then we get the second line which is called line of residual. The slope rate of this line equals to $-k_a/2.303$, and then k_a is calculated.

3. Absolute bioavailability

Bioavailability refers to the degree to which or rate at which a drug or other substance is absorbed or becomes available at the site of physiological activity after administration. Bioavailability includes absolute bioavailability F and relative bioavailability F_r. Preparation for intravenous injection is usually as the control preparation of absolute bioavailability used for study of Raw Material Medicines and novel dosage forms.

$$F = \frac{AUC_{(po)}/Dose_{(po)}}{AUC_{(iv)}/Dose_{(iv)}} \times 100\% \tag{7-15}$$

Each subject should administrate the control preparation and thereference preparation at different time, respectively. The two－period Cross－over design is useful to counteract effects of time on results. Rabbits were randomly divided into two groups and were administered with different preparations because of time available.

Materials andinstruments

1. Materials

All of the chemicals employed in the experiment are analytical grade unless otherwise specified. Acetaminophen tablets (300mg), Acetaminophen injection (100mg/ml), normal saline, 1% heparin sodium, 10% perchloric acid, methanol (chromatographic grade).

2. Instruments

HPLC system, vortexer, centrifuge machine, syringe injector (50ml), wooden ton for fixing rabbits, infrared lamp, gavage device, blade, beaker.

3. Animals

Rabbits weighting about 2. 5kg are fasted for 12 hours with free access to drinking water.

Procedures

1. Determination of the standard curves

(1) Preparation of the standard curve

A stock solution of 2000μg/ml acetaminophen was prepared by dissolving acetaminophen in methanol – water (50 : 50). A series of standard solutions were prepared by adding 0. 1ml, 0. 2ml, 0. 5ml, 1ml, 2ml, 5ml, 10ml of stock solution to 10ml volumetric flasks.

A series of standard solutions (4 ~ 400μg/ml) were prepared by adding 20μl of solutions above to tubes with 80μl blank blood plasma. 100μl of 10% perchloric acid was added to tubes, then mix it and centrifuge it at 12000r/min for 10minutes. 20μl of supernatant is removed for analysis, and chromatogram and peak area are recorded. Standard curve equation of peak area (A) versus concentration (C, mg/ml) was analyzed.

(2) the HPLC method

Thechromatographic column: ODS C_{18} (150mm × 4. 6mm, 5mm)

The mobile phase: methanol – water (30 : 70)

The wavelength of determination: 272nm

The flow rate: 1. 0ml/min

The column temperature: 30℃

The volume of the injection: 20ml

2. Sampling

(1) Administration design

Six rabbits are weighed and divided into two groups randomly. The first cycle: the first group is administrated intragastricly with test product A (acetaminophen is dissolved and diluted with 40ml normal saline); the second group is administrated intravenously with reference product B (dose is 100mg/kg). After rinsed, the second cycle: the first group is administrated intravenously with reference product. The second group is administrated intragastricly. 0. 5ml blank blood is withdrawn from vein of the edge of the ear prior to each administration and placed into EP tubes coated with heparin.

(2) Blood collection

After administration, 0. 5ml of blood will be sampled into EP tubes coated with heparin at the intervals 0. 25h, 0. 5, 1, 1. 5, 2, 3, 4, 6, 8, 10, 12 and 24 hours, and centrifuge it at 3000r/min for

10 minutes, thenthe upper plasma is taken for analysis.

3. Determination Method of acetaminophen blood concentration

100μl blood samples are added to EP tubes with 100μl of 10% perchloric acid, then mix it and centrifuge it at 12000r/min for 10 minutes. Then 20μl of supernatant is removed for analysis, and chromatogram and peak area are recorded.

4. Data processing

(1) The Standard Curve of acetaminophen

Fill the Tab. 7 – 1, and the standard curve can be obtained by linear regression.

Tab. 7 – 1　The standard curve of acetaminophen

C(μg/ml)
A

Regression equation: C =

Regression coefficient: r =

Linear range:　　–　　μg/ml.

(2) Data followingintravenous injection

Fill the Tab. 7 – 2 with data obtained followingintravenous injection.

Tab. 7 – 2　Data of intravenous injection

t(hours)	0.25	0.5	1.0	1.5	2.0	3.0	4.0	6.0	8.0	10	12	24
A												
C												

The parameters k, $t_{1/2}$, C_0, V, Cl and $AUC_{(iv)}$ are estimated by using the related equations in the Introduction.

(3) Data following oral administration

Fill the Tab. 7 – 3 with data obtained followingoral administration.

Tab. 7 – 3　Data of oral administration

t(hours)	A	C	$\ln C$	C'	$C' - C$	$\ln(C' - C)$
0.25						
0.5						
1.0						
1.5						
2.0						
3.0						
4.0						
6.0						
8.0						
10						
12						
24						

The parameters$k$, k_a, $t_{1/2}$, and $AUC_{(po)}$ are estimated by using the related equations in the Introduction.

(4) Absolute bioavailability(F)

Absolute bioavailability(F) is calculated using Eq. (7 – 15).

(5) Pharmacokinetics parameters

Fill the Tab. 7 – 4 with data obtained followingoral administration and intravenous injection.

Tab. 7 – 4 Pharmacokinetic parameters

	k (h^{-1})	$t_{1/2}$ (h)	k_a (h^{-1})	V (ml)	Cl(ml/h) (kV)	AUC (h · μg/ml)	Cl_s(ml/h) (X_0/AUC)
i. v. oral ad.							

(6) Summary

Calculate the mean value and standard deviation by mathematical statistic analysis of data, plot lnC versus t to obtain pharmacokinetics parameters, fill Tab. 9 – 5 with these data and write out the expression of a concentration – time relationship according to Eq. (7 – 1) and Eq. (7 – 8).

Tab. 7 – 5 Plasma concentration and pharmacokinetic parameters(n = 6)

t(hours)	intravenous injection							oral administration						
	1	2	3	4	5	6	$\bar{x} \pm s$	1	2	3	4	5	6	$\bar{x} \pm s$
0.25														
0.5														
1.0														
1.5														
2.0														
3.0														
4.0														
6.0														
8.0														
10														
12														
24														
k(h^{-1})														
AUC (h · μg/ml)														
F(%)														

Experimental Guidelines

Requirements for preview

1. To review the chapters in pharmacological experiments concerning procedures(intravenous administration, oral administration and vein on the ear border of rabbit).

2. To review theestimation of pharmacokinetics parameters.

3. To be familiar with the basic operations of HPLC.

4. To learn the determination principle of acetaminophen in plasma, and the method of data processing.

Precautions

1. For oral administration, fix the rabbit firstly and insert the wood - made mouth - gag into the mouth of the rabbit. A tablet is put into throat carefully by bend pincer and rinsed into stomach with some water.

2. For intravenous injection, fix the rabbit into a special box and make the vein in the back and external ear seen clearly by cutting the fur. Secondly, hold the tip of the ear with the thumb and middle finger and support under the vein with the forefinger of the left hand. Thirdly, insert needle into the vein from the tip at an angle of 5° and fix the needle inside by pressing it outside with thumb, fore finger, and middle finger of the left hand in case the needle goes out of the vein when the rabbit moves its head.

3. To avoid blood coagulation, the test tube should be soaked evenly with 1% heparin sodium in advance and put into an oven at 80℃ to dry.

4. Hemolysis is caused by erythrocytes rupture and substance such as hemoglobin are released into plasma. Because the concentration of many substance in plasma is different from that in erythrocytes hemolysis will effect on accuracy of determination. During sampling not squeeze vascular forcibly and keep blood flowing into test tubes slowly in case of hemolysis.

Questions

1. Please explain conditions and procedures of data processing using the method of residual.

2. What methods for calculation of Cl_s are introduced in the experiment? Please explain their advantages and limitations.

References

1. Zhang JR. Pharmaceutical Analysis in Vivo[M]. Chemical Industry Press. 2002.

2. Liang WQ. Biopharmaceutics and Pharmacokinetics [M]. People's Medical Publishing House. 2003.

扫码“学一学”

实验八　药物动力学单隔室模型模拟实验

【目的与要求】

1. **掌握**　用模拟实验的数据计算药物动力学参数的方法。

2. **了解**　体外单隔室模拟实验的原理和方法。

【基本概念和实验原理】

一、血药浓度法

若药物在体内的分布符合单室模型特征，且按表观一级动力学从体内消除，则快速静脉注射时，体内药物随时间变化的表达式为：

$$C = C_0 e^{-kt} \tag{8-1}$$

对数表达式为：

$$\ln C = -kt + \ln C_0 \tag{8-2}$$

式中，C_0 为静注后最初的血药浓度，C 为 t 时间的血药浓度。以 $\ln C$ 对 t 作图，可得一条直线。由直线的斜率和截距求出表观一级消除速度常数 k 和消除半衰期 $t_{1/2}$。

$$t_{1/2} = 0.693/k \tag{8-3}$$

$$V = \frac{X_0}{C_0} \tag{8-4}$$

二、尿排泄速率

药物从体内排泄的途径主要为经肾排泄，其次为由肾外途径排泄。药物服用后，如果有较多药物从尿中排泄，并且假定药物经肾排泄符合一级速率过程，则可用尿药排泄数据求算药动学参数。

设 X_u 为原形消除于尿中的药物量；k_e、k_{nr} 分别为肾排泄和非肾途径消除的表观一级速度常数。于是消除速度常数

$$k = k_e + k_{nr} \tag{8-5}$$

1. **速率法**　尿药速率可表示为：

$$\frac{dX_u}{dt} = K_e X \tag{8-6}$$

由 8-1 式可得

$$X = X_0 \cdot e^{-kt} \tag{8-7}$$

将公式 8-7 代入 8-6，可得：

$$\frac{dX_u}{dt} = K_e X_0 \cdot e^{-kt} \tag{8-8}$$

两边取对数可得：

$$\log \frac{dX_u}{dt} = \log k_e X_0 - \frac{kt}{2.303} \qquad (8-9)$$

上式中，X_0为给药剂量。由于用实验方法求出的尿药排泄速度不是瞬时速度（dX_u/dt），而是一段有限时间内的平均速度 $\Delta X_u/\Delta t$，则用 $\Delta X_u/\Delta t$ 代替上式中的 dX_u/dt，以集尿间隔内的中点时间时间对平均速度的对数作图为一条直线，其斜率为 $-k/2.303$，与血药浓度法所求的斜率相同。

2. 亏量法　待排泄药量的经时过程表达式为：

$$\ln(X_u^{\infty} - X_u) = -kt + lnX_u^{\infty} \qquad (8-10)$$

式中，X_u^{∞} 为尿中原形药物排泄量，（$X_u^{\infty} - X_u$）为待排泄原形药物量，或称为亏量。以亏量的对数对时间作图为一条直线，通过其斜率和截距可求得 k 和 k_e。

三、实验原理

单室模拟装置为带有两支管的三角烧瓶，如图 8－1 所示，烧瓶为模拟体循环系统，其中的试液为“血液”。当把药物（酚红）注入烧瓶中后，用恒流泵将水以一定的流速注入烧瓶中模拟人正常水分的摄入，A、B 两管可分别看作非肾排泄和肾排泄两种消除途径，药物不断地从 A、B 两管中清除。其中控制支管 A 的液体连续滴出作为非肾排泄途径；控制 B 管液体连续流出作为肾排泄途径，该液体被视为“尿液”。

由于在生理条件下，经肾排泄途径产生的尿液会在膀胱中储存，在达到一定量后才会被排出体外。因此，为了更好地模拟体内药物经肾排泄途径消除的过程，在 B 支管下方放置一个 50ml 的量杯模拟膀胱，用于储存一段时间内通过肾排泄途径产生的“尿液”。

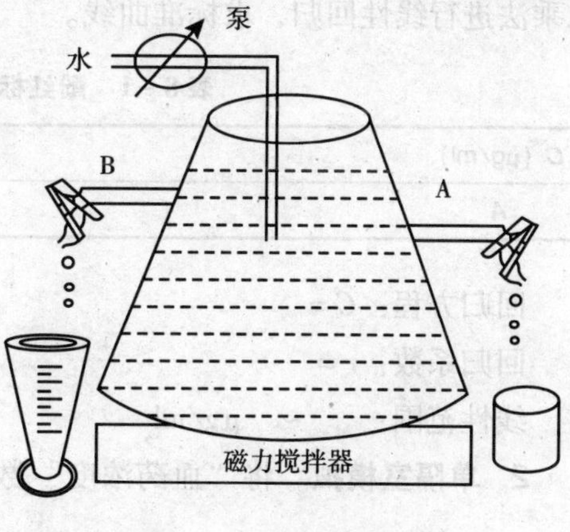

图 8－1　模拟装置示意图

【材料与仪器】

1. 材料　0.1% 酚红试液，1% Na_2CO_3溶液，0.2mol/L NaOH 溶液等。

2. 仪器　恒流泵，磁力搅拌器，752 型分光光度计，三角烧瓶（带两个支管），橡皮管，夹子，搅拌子，量杯，试管等。

【实验内容】

一、酚红标准曲线的制备

精密称取酚红 100mg，置 1000ml 容量瓶内，加 1% Na_2CO_3溶液至刻度，配成100μg/ml 的储备液，分别吸取 0.5，1，1.5，2，2.5，3ml 的储备液，加水至 10ml，得一系列标准液。照定量方法项下测定酚红的吸收度并绘制标准曲线。

扫码“看一看”

二、单隔室模拟操作方法

1. 单隔室模拟　将约 250ml 的水倒入三角烧瓶中，开动磁力搅拌器。用恒流泵以每分钟约 8ml 的流速将水注入烧瓶中，搅拌 10 分钟。用橡皮管与夹子控制支管中的液体连续滴出，支管 A 的流速为每分钟 2ml，支管 B 的流速为每分钟 4ml。保证三角烧瓶内液面始终高于 B 管出水孔。

2. 取样 用移液管将烧瓶中的水取出 10ml，然后移取 0.1% 酚红供试液 10ml，加入烧瓶中并记时，以后每隔 10 分钟从烧瓶中取 0.5ml 试液作为“血药样品”，同时撤离 B 管下方量杯并立即更换量杯重新收集下一时间段的“尿液”。记录撤离下来的量杯内的“尿液”体积，从中收集 0.5ml 量杯内储存的液体作为“尿药样品”。

三、定量方法

取 0.5ml “血药样品”（或“尿药样品”），加入 0.2mol/L NaOH 溶液 5ml，在波长 550nm 处测定酚红的吸收度并计算浓度。

四、数据处理

1. 酚红的标准曲线 将酚红的标准溶液的浓度及相应的吸收度填入表 8-1，并按最小二乘法进行线性回归，求标准曲线。

表 8-1 酚红标准溶液的浓度及相应的吸收度

C (μg/ml)	
A	

回归方程：$C=$

回归系数：$r=$

线性范围： ~ μg/ml

2. 单隔室模拟 将“血药浓度”数据和“尿排泄”数据记录于表 8-2、表 8-3。

表 8-2 酚红的“血药浓度”数据

取样时间（分钟）	10	20	30	40	50	60	70	80
吸收度								
浓度								

试求算 k，$t_{1/2}$，V。

表 8-3 酚红“尿排泄”数据

时间（分钟）	10	20	30	40	50	60	70	80	300
V (ml)									
A									
C									
ΔX_u									
X_u									
Δt									
t_{middle}									

（1）速率法 根据尿药速率法公式求算 k，$t_{1/2}$ 和 k_e。

（2）亏量法　以300分钟时的 X_u 作为尿中原形药物排泄总量 X_u^∞，根据亏量法原理求算 k，$t_{1/2}$ 和 k_e。

【实验指导】

一、预习要求

1. 学习　体外单隔室模拟试验的原理。
2. 了解　酚红含量测定的方法。

二、操作要点和注意事项

1. 保证三角烧瓶内液面始终高于 B 管出水孔，使支管 B 可连续流出液体，以模拟药物以肾排泄方式从体内消除。

2. 撤离 B 管下方量杯后，应立即放置新的量杯收集下一时间点的“尿药样品”，使 B 管流出的液体均流入到量杯内，保证样品数据的准确性。

3. 酚红的测定中，应以 0.2mol/l 的 NaOH 溶液为空白对照。

扫码“练一练”

三、思考题

1. 本实验中的模拟装置有何意义？操作中应注意哪些问题？
2. 本实验中介绍了哪两种通过尿排泄数据求算药动学参数的方法？试比较两者的优缺点。
3. 取样总时间、取样间隔、酚红加入量、恒流泵流速、支管滴速等因素对实验结果（如 k 值）有无影响？

参考文献

1. 屠锡德，张钧寿，朱家壁，等．药剂学［M］．北京：人民卫生出版社，2002.
2. 朱家壁译．生物药剂学［M］．北京：人民卫生出版社，1987.

Experiment 8　Simulation of One－Compartment Model

Purposes

1. To master theestimation methods for pharmacokinetics parameters using data of simulation experiment.

2. To be familiar with the basic procedures in thesimulation of the one－compartment model.

Introduction

1. Drug concentration in the plasma

Following rapid intravenous injection of a drug that distributes in the body according to a one－compartment model and is eliminated by apparent first－order kinetics, the time course of plasma concentration of drug is given by

$$C = C_0 e^{-kt} \qquad (8-1)$$

Therefore,

$$\ln C = -kt + \ln C_0 \qquad (8-2)$$

where C_0 is the drug concentration in plasma immediately after injection. C is the drug concentration in the plasma at any time t after injection. Eq. (8 – 2) indicates that a plot of log C versus t will be linear. Hence the elimination rate constant and the elimination half life can be estimated from the plot of log plasma drug concentration versus time.

$$t_{1/2} = 0.693/k \quad (8-3)$$

$$V = \frac{X_0}{C_0} \quad (8-4)$$

C_0 could be obtained by the extrapolation of the log C versus t plot to time zero. This intercept, C_0 can be used in the calculation of the apparent volume of distribution(V).

2. The rate method of urinary excretion

It is sometimes possible to consider the elimination kinetics of a drug from urinary excretion data if some – extent of the unchanged drug is subject to urinary excretion. In this calculation the excretion rate of drug is assumed to be first. Consider a drug eliminated from the body partly by renal excretion and partly by nonrenal processes such as biotransformation and biliary excretion. The elimination rate constant k is the sum of the individual rate constants that characterize the parallel elimination processes. Thus

$$k = k_e + k_{nr} \quad (8-5)$$

where k_e is the apparent first – order rate constant for renal excretion and k_{nr} is the sum of all other apparent first – order rate constants for drug elimination by nonrenal pathways, respectively.

(1) The urinary excretion rates method

The excretion rate of unchanged drug, dXu/dt, can be defined as

$$\frac{dX_u}{dt} = K_e X \quad (8-6)$$

where X is the amount of drug in the body at time$t$ and X_u is the cumulative amounts of eliminated and unchanged drug in the urine.

We can get Eq. (8 – 7) by deriving Eq. (8 – 1)

$$X = X_0 \cdot e^{-kt} \quad (8-7)$$

Combine Eq. (8 – 6) and Eq. (8 – 7), therefore,

$$\frac{dX_u}{dt} = K_e X_0 \cdot e^{-kt} \quad (8-8)$$

Calculate Eq. (8 – 8) using log at both side, then:

$$\log \frac{dX_u}{dt} = \log k_e X_0 - \frac{kt}{2.303} \quad (8-9)$$

These experimentally determined excretion rates are obviously not instantaneous rates (i. e., dX_u/dt), but are average rates over a finite time period (i. e. $\Delta Xu/\Delta t$). However, the average excretion rate closely approximates the instantaneous excretion rate at the midpoint of the urine collection period if Δt approaches zero. A logarithmic plot of average excretion rate of unchanged drug versus time is linear, with a slope of $-k/2.303$. This slope is the same as that obtained from a nature log arithmic plot of drug concentration in plasma versus time. In addition, k_e can be calculated from the intercept of the line.

(2) The Sigma – minus method

The time course of amount of unchanged drug remaining to be excreted (A. R. E.) is given by

$$\ln(X_u^{\infty} - X_u) = -kt + \ln X_u^{\infty} \quad (8-10)$$

Where X_u^{∞} is the amount of unchanged drug ultimately eliminated in the urine, ($X_u^{\infty} - X_u$) is the amount of unchanged drug remaining to be encreted (A. R. E.), a plot of log A. R. E. versus time is linear with a slope equal to $-k$ and a intercept of X_u^{∞}.

3. Principles of the experiment

The simulated device of the one – compartment model is the triangular flask with two branches, as shown in Fig. 8 – 1. The flask is regarded as the systemic circulatory system, and the solution in it as "blood". After water is placed into the flask with drug (phenol red), water is continued to pump into the flask at a constant flow rate for the simulation of water intake. Drug was assumed to eliminate from two branches, represented by "renal excretion" (branch B in the Fig. 8 – 1) and by "nonrenal processes" (branch A in the Fig. 8 – 1), respectively.

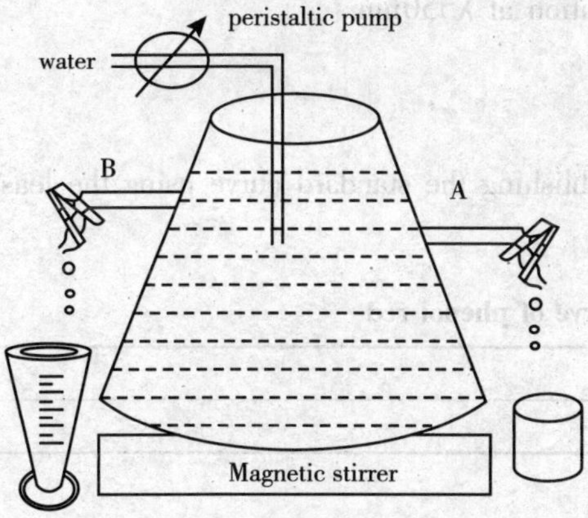

Fig. 8 – 1　Simulation for the One – Compartment Model

Since the urine produced by the renal excretion pathway is stored in the bladder under physiological conditions, it will be excreted after reaching a certain amount. Therefore, in order to better simulate the elimination of drugs in the body through the renal excretion pathway, a 50ml measuring cup was placed under the B – branch to simulate the bladder, which was used to store the "urine" produced by the renal excretion route for a period of time.

Materials andinstruments

1. Materials

All of the chemicals employed in this experiment are analytical grade unless otherwise specified. 0.1% phenol red solution, 1% sodium carbonate solution, 0.2mol/L sodium hydroxide solution.

2. Instruments

Peristaltic pump, magnetic stirrer, spectrophotometer model 752, triangular flask with two branches, rubber hose, clamp, magnetic stir bar measuring cup, test tube.

Procedures

1. Preparation of standard curve

A stock solution (100μg/ml of phenol) was prepared by dissolving 100mg in 1000ml of 1% sodium carbonate. A series of standard solutions (5 – 30μg/ml) were prepared by diluting the initial stock solution with water. 5ml of 0.2mol/L NaOH was added to each 0.5ml of standard solution and mixed. Determine the absorbance of the resulting solution at λ550nm.

2. Simulation of One – Compartment Model

(1) Simulation of one – compartment model

250ml of water in the triangular flask is stirred on a magnetic stirrer. Water is pumped into the flask at flow rate of 8ml/min by use of a peristaltic pump and is stirred for 10 minutes. The liquid in the branch pipe was continuously discharged by a rubber tube and a clip. The flow rate of the branch pipe A was 2ml per minute, and the flow rate of the branch pipe B was 4ml per minute. Ensure that the liquid level in the triangular beaker is always higher than the B tube outlet.

(2) Sampling

Take 10ml of water from the flask and add an equal volume of 0.1% phenol red into the flask. At 10 minutes intervals, take 0.5ml of water from the flask as the observed "plasma" sample while evacuate the measuring cup below the B tube. Replace the measuring cup immediately to collect the "urine" for the next period of time. Record the volume of "urine" in the evacuated measuring cup and withraw 0.5ml liquid stored in it as a "urine sample".

3. Determination of phenol red

5ml of 0.2mol/L NaOH was added to each 0.5ml of "plasma" sample (or "urine" sample) and mixed. Measure the absorbance of the resulting solution at λ550nm.

4. Data processing

(1) The Stand curve of phenol red

Fill Tab. 8-1 with the absorbance readings for establishing the standard curve using the least-square method.

Tab. 8-1 The standard curve of phenol red

C(μg/ml)	
A	

Regression equation: *C* =

Regression coefficient: *r* =

Linear range: -   μg/ml.

(2) Simulation of One - Compartment Model

Fill Tab. 8-2 and Tab. 8-3 with data obtained following sampling.

Tab. 8-2 The "plasma" concentration data

t (minutes)	10	20	30	40	50	60	70	80
A								
C(μg/ml)								

The parameters k, $t_{1/2}$, V are estimated by using the related equations in the Introduction.

Tab. 8-3 The "urinary" excretion data

t (minutes)	10	20	30	40	50	60	70	80	300
V(ml)									
A									
C									
ΔX_u									
X_u									
Δt									
t_{middle}									

① The method of urinary excretion rates

The parameters k, $t_{1/2}$ and k_e are estimated by using the related equations in the Introduction.

② The Sigma – minus method

If the "drug" is completely eliminated from the system in 300minutes, X_u at 300minutes is regarded as X_u^{∞}. The parameters k, $t_{1/2}$ and k_e are estimated by using the related equations in the Introduction.

Experimental Guidelines

Requirements for preview

1. To learn the principle of the simulation of one – compartment model.
2. To know the determination of phenol red.

Precautions

1. Ensure that the liquid level in the conical flask is always higher than the B tube outlet, so that the branch B can continuously flow out of the liquid to simulate the elimination of the drug from the body by renal excretion.
2. After evacuating the measuring cup below the B tube, a new measuring cup should be placed immediately to collect the "urinary drug sample" for the next period of time, so that the liquid flowing out of the B tube completely flows into the measuring cup to ensure the accuracy of the sample data.
3. The blank solution should be 0. 2mol/L sodium hydroxide solution.

Questions

1. What are the implications in the designed flask and the two branches in thisexperiment? Which attentions should be focused?
2. What methods for the estimation of the parameters are introduced in the experimont? Please explain their advantages and limitations?
3. Do the total sampling time, sampling interval, amount of phenol red, flow rate of constant flow pump and dropping speed of the branch affect the estimated parameter k?

References

1. Tu Xide, Zhang Junshou, Zhu Jiabi, etal. Pharmaceutics[M]. People's Medical Publishing House. 2002.
2. Zhu Jiabi. Biopharmaceutics[M]. People's Medical Publishing House. 1987.

扫码“学一学”

扫码“看一看”

实验九　药物动力学实验数据的处理

【目的要求】

1. **掌握**　非线性回归方法在药物动力学实验数据处理中的应用。
2. **了解**　模型分析方法中线性与非线性模型概念；模型线性回归和非线性回归方法。

【基本概念与原理】

一、模型的应用

数学模型在科学研究、社会生活等方面具有重要的作用，广泛应用于各类观察或数据的定量分析，主要用于分析实验数据、验证假设、定量预测。随着计算机及相应技术在各个领域的广泛应用，人类借助数学模型解决问题的能力得到了很大的提高。同样，模型在药学领域尤其是药物体内配置研究具有极大的价值。

二、数学模型分类

数学模型通常可以划分为两类：线性模型与非线性模型。在线性模型中，因变量通常等于自变量与各自参数乘积之和。例如，代表某一直线方程式：

$$Y = A + B \cdot X \tag{9-1}$$

在该方程式中，Y是因变量，X是自变量，A是截距，B是斜率。

其他常见的线性模型中函数关系有多项式 $Y = A_1 + A_2X + A_3X^2 + A_4X^3$，多元函数式 $Y = A_1 + A_2X_1 + A_3X_2 + A_4X_3$。

在表达线性模型的函数关系式中，所有的参数仅仅作为自变量的系数出现。然而，在代表非线性模型中变量关系的函数关系式中，至少一个参数是以自变量的非系数形式出现，例如，$C = C_0e^{-kt}$，$C = Ae^{-\alpha t} + Be^{-\beta t}$，$\nu = \dfrac{V_{\max}C}{K_m + C}$。

由此可见，经典药物动力学研究方法与非线性模型密切相关。

三、回归分析

回归分析（regression）系指研究自变量与因变量之间非确定性因果关系的方法。相对于线性模型和非线性模型，在研究各自的变量之间关系时，应该分别采用线性回归分析（linear regression）和非线性回归分析（nonlinear regression）。

1. （一元）线性回归 $Y = A + BX$　直线线性回归的目的就是根据若干个观测（X_i，Y_i，$i = 1, ..., n$），找出描述两个变量X、Y之间关系的直线回归方程$Y = A + BX$，实际上就是用回归直线拟合散点图中的各实测值点。常用的方法有最小二乘法线性回归（Least Square Linear Regression），使该直线与各点的纵向垂直距离最小，也就是使实测值Y_i与回归直线得

到的计算值 Y^* 之差的残差、剩余平方和（$\sum_{i=1}^{n}(Y-Y^*)^2$）达到最小。

因此，求回归方程 $Y^*=A+BX$ 的问题，即成为求 $\sum_{i=1}^{n}(Y-Y^*)^2$ 取得最小值时 A 和 B 的问题。A 为回归直线截距，B 为回归直线斜率，也称回归系数。

然而，采用线性回归方程时，所分析的实测值必须具有正态分布（a Gaussian distribution）的性质，而且假定所有点的方差（σ^2）相同。这是进行线性回归分析方法条件之一。在进行药物动力学实验数据的分析处理之中，即使面对是非线性模型，但限于计算技术的制约，为简便起见，可以通过数据变换，将自变量与因变量之间非线性关系变成线性关系。例如，将 $C=C_0e^{-kt}$ 里边取对数，变成 $\log C=\log C_0-kt$，以及将 $\nu=\frac{V_{\max}C}{K_m+C}$ 变换成 $\frac{1}{\nu}=\frac{1}{V_{\max}}+\frac{K_m}{V_{\max}}\cdot\frac{1}{C}$。然后，通过最小二乘法线性回归进行数据分析，求取模型的各项参数。但是，将非线性数据转变为线性数据，通常会违背上述采用线性回归分析的条件，误导数据偏差。因此，最终导致参数估算值准确性不高。

同时，许多非线性模型是不能通过数据变换为线性模型。例如，单室口服模型与双室静注模型等，至少为两指数项值之和（或差）。这时根本无法采用线性回归方法。需要进一步指出的是，药物动力学实验数据处理中，经常采用的残数法与尿药速率法或尿药亏量法皆为主观决断下舍去部分数据，采用局部数据进行线性回归分析，造成模型参数估计值准确性和可靠性很差。

2. 非线性回归　非线性回归方法更具有通用性。在确定代表非线性模型的自变量与因变量之间函数关系 Y = F（X）之后，非线性回归方法根据所提供的实验数据和函数关系（即方程式，包括代数方程式和微分方程式），通过迭代方法（带入选定的参数初始值），最终选定的参数值应该使得根据此参数值和函数关系计算得到的拟合曲线和实验数据最接近，或者说，实验数据点与这条曲线的垂直距离平方和为最小化（least square）。同时，也就是讲满足了所谓最佳嵌合（best fit）条件之一。

通过迭代方法计算函数参数的常见计算方法有单纯形法（Nelder – Mead Simplex）和高斯 – 牛顿法（Levenberg – Marquardt Modification）。

四、非线性回归分析在药动学实验数据处理中的应用

1. 计算机程序 3p97 及介绍　3p97 与 GraphPad Prism ®

2. 利用非线性回归程序进行药物血药浓度 – 时间数据嵌合

3. 隔室模型研究方法　药物动力学主要是定量研究药物经各种途径进入机体的吸收、分布、代谢和排泄的经时变化过程，同时也探讨人和动物体内相应药理、临床及毒副作用的经时变化过程。研究中有必要理解接受药物输入的生物系统的解剖学和生理学特征，以及模型的概念和限制条件。人们主要将用于表征药物浓度 – 时间关系的模型分为隔室模型和生理模型，对隔室模型有较早的认识与运用。借助化学动力学理论和隔室概念，隔室模型方法从而能够确定体内药物数量或浓度与时间的关系。最常用的隔室模型有如下的单室模型和双室模型：

MODEL 1. One-compartment open model, Ⅳ injection.

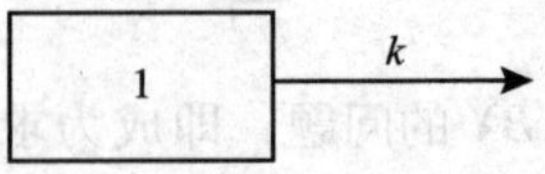

MODEL 2. One-compartment open model with first-order absorption.

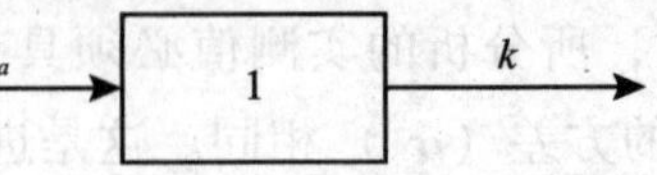

MODEL 3. Two-compartment open model, Ⅳ injection.

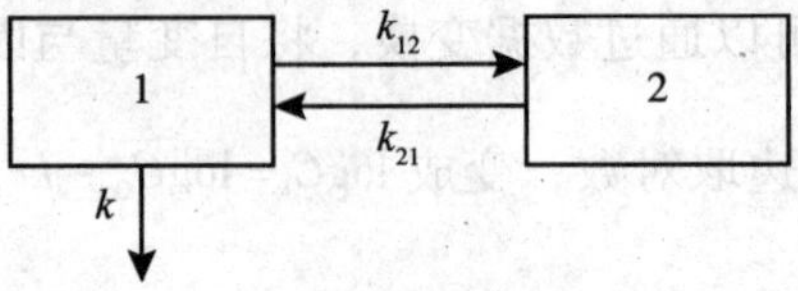

MODEL 4. Two-compartment open model with first-order absorption.

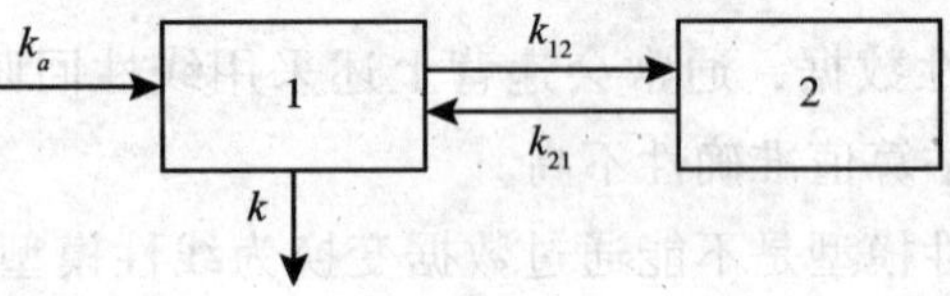

对应上述模型的、表达药物浓度与时间的关系如下：

$$C = \frac{X_0}{V_d}e^{-kt} \tag{9-2}$$

$$C = \frac{k_a F X_0}{V_d(k_a - k)}(e^{-kt} - e^{-k_a t}) \tag{9-3}$$

$$C = Ae^{-\alpha t} + Be^{-\beta t} \tag{9-4}$$

$$C = Ne^{-k_a t} + Le^{-\alpha t} + Me^{-\beta t} \tag{9-5}$$

4. 模型选择

（1）作图比较　对于静脉注射后获得的血药浓度数据，如果 $\log C$ 对时间作图具有线性，这样可能判断此药物体内具有单室模型特征。否则，应属于多室模型。然而，此方法有主观猜测性问题。

（2）根据统计学信息

a. 残差平方和（SS）

$$SS = \sum_{i=1}^{n}(Y_i - Y_i^*)^2 \tag{9-6}$$

b. 回归系数（R^2）

$$R^2 = 1 - \frac{\sum_{i=1}^{n}(Y_i - Y_i^*)^2}{\sum_{i=1}^{n}Y_i^2} \tag{9-7}$$

c. 赤池信息矩（AIC）

$$AIC = N \cdot \ln(SS) + 2M \tag{9-8}$$

上式中，SS 为残差平方和，N 是实验数据组组数，M 为所采用的模型公式中参数个数。

对模型选择而言，SS 和 AIC 数值越小，拟合效果越好，拟合数值越接进实验数据。鉴于考虑模型中公式参数个数的影响，AIC 为适宜模型选择的指标。

五、非线性回归分析在药动学实验数据处理中的应用

1. 计算机程序 3P97 及介绍演示。

2. 利用非线性回归程序进行药物血药浓度－时间数据嵌合，实验数据如下。

（1）静注给药 A（剂量：100mg）后，测定血药浓度如表 9－1。

表 9－1　静注药物 A 血药浓度－时间关系

T（小时）	0.25	0.5	0.75	1.0	1.25	1.5	2	3	4
C（mg/ml）	58.98	54.10	49.59	46.65	43.38	41.02	36.73	30.58	26.54
T（小时）	6	8	10	12	16	20	24	36	48
C（mg/ml）	22.20	19.23	17.41	15.59	12.71	10.36	8.45	4.57	2.48

（2）静注给药 B（剂量：100mg）后，测定血药浓度如表 9－2。

表 9－2　静注药物 B 血药浓度－时间关系

T（小时）	0.25	0.5	0.75	1.0	2.0	3.0	4.0	6.0	8.0	10.0	14	18	24
C（mg/ml）	11.62	10.31	10.96	9.70	9.55	7.65	7.45	5.34	4.70	3.43	2.29	1.30	0.71

（3）口服给药 B（剂量：200mg）后，测定血药浓度如表 9－3。

表 9－3　口服药物 B 血药浓度－时间关系

T（小时）	0.2	0.4	0.6	0.8	1.0	1.5	2.5	4.0	5.0	6.0	7.0
C（mg/ml）	1.65	2.33	2.55	2.51	2.40	2.00	1.27	0.66	0.39	0.25	0.15

3. 数据处理记录、处理与模型选择　包括如下内容。

（1）参数估算值，标准差（误），95% 置信区间。

（2）实测值（Yi）与计算值（Yi＊）。

（3）实测值（Yi）与计算值（Yi＊）之间残差值。

（4）实测值与计算值之间残差值对时间作图。

（5）残差平方和（SS）。

（6）拟合度（R^2）。

（7）AIC。

【实验指导】

思考题

1. 药物动力学数据模型分析如果采用残数法，此方法有何严重缺限？

2. 残数法中采用的是哪种回归方法？

3. 对数据模型分析来说，模型判断的依据有哪些？最重要的依据是哪个？

4. 对模型判断来说，为什么 AIC 比 SS 更重要？

扫码“练一练”

参考文献

1. Bourne D. *Mathematical Modeling of Pharmacokinetic Data*[M]. Lancaster, PA: Technomic Publishing, 1995.

2. Gibaldi M. *Biopharmaceutics and Clinical Pharmacokinetics*. 3rd ed[M]. Philadelphia, PA: Lea and Febiger, 1984.

3. Jambhekar S and Breen PJ. *Basic Pharmacokinetics*. 2nd ed[M]. Philadelphia, PA: Pharmaceutical Press, 2012.

4. Bonate PL. *Pharmacokinetic – Pharmacodynamic Modeling and Simulation*[M]. New York, NY: Springer, 2006.

Experiment 9 Fitting Data into a Pharmacokinetic Model

Purposes

1. To understand the application of nonlinear regression in pharmacoketic model.

2. to be familiar with the concept of statistical linear and nonlinear models, and the linear and nonlinear regressions.

Introduction

1. Models represent the system under study.

Mathematical models are very vital in many areas such as scientific research and social observation, and they have wide applications in various quantitative analyses including data analysis, validation of hypothesis, and quantitative prediction. With widespread availability of computers and the computation technologies, enhanced capability in the utilization of modeling – based scientific investigation towards problem solving occurs. Similarly, modeling markedly contributes to the insight into *in vivo* drug disposition.

2. Mathematical models are generally divided into two categories, ie, linear and nonlinear models. In linear models, dependent variable can be expressed as the sum of products of the independent *variable* and *parameters*(coefficients). For example, a straight line is defined by the equation

$$Y = A + B \cdot X \quad (9-1)$$

where Y is the dependent variable, X is the independent variable, A is the Y – intercept and B is the slope.

It also be represented by the polynomial function such as $Y = A_1 + A_2X + A_3X^2 + A_4X^3$ and a function of several variables $Y = A_1 + A_2X_1 + A_3X_2 + A_4X_3$.

In nonlinear models if expressed by the equation, at least one of the parameters appears as other than a coefficient. For example, $C = C_0e^{-kt}$, $C = Ae^{-\alpha t} + Be^{-\beta t}$, $\nu = \frac{V_{\max}C}{K_m + C}$

3. Regression

Regression analysis is a statistical technique that defines the functional relationship between two variables. In characterization of the functional relationship between variables, linear and nonlinear regressionsare employed.

(1) Linear regression $Y = A + BX$

Simple linear regression analysis is a statistical technique that, based on $(X_i, Y_i, i = 1, \ldots, n)$, defines the functional relationship between two variables, X and Y, ie, the "best – fitting" straight line. The common method is least squares linear regression. It applies to the solution of relations where the function of Y is linear in the parameter. A plot of Y vs. X data rarely exactly fits a straight line. The line does not go exactly through all of the poins. A "good" line, however, should come "close" to the experimental points. It is defined that the best straight line describing the relation of Y and X as the line that minimizes the sum of squares of the vertical distances of each point from the fitted line. The definition of "sum of squares of the vertical distances of each oint from the fitted line" is written mathematically as ($\sum_{i=1}^{n} (Y - Y^*)^2$), where Y represents the experimental points and Y^* represents the corresponding points on the fitted line. The line constructed according to this definition is called the least squares line only if we we believe that the true relationship between Y and X is linear. The slope of intercept of the least squares line can be calculated from the observation data.

However, if applying least squares method, all of the observation data must indicate a Gaussian distribution. In the analysis of data obtained in pharmacokinetics study, we often encounter nonlinear model and have limited access to the computation technology in the past years. For simplicity, data transformation can allow the conversion of nonlinearity into linearity between data. For example, taking the natural log on both side of $C = C_0e^{-kt}$ permits transformation to a linear equation $\log C = \log C_0 - kt$. Similarly, $v = \frac{V_{max}C}{K_m + C}$ is transformed to $\frac{1}{v} = \frac{1}{V_{max}} + \frac{K_m}{V_{max}} \cdot \frac{1}{C}$. Then we apply least squares regression to fit the "best – fitted" to data. But, the transformation often results in distorted, or biased data and corresponding inaccuracy in the parameter estimation. Therefore, this is not recommended.

In addition, it is usual that many nonlinear models can not transformed to linear ones. For instance, as in the cases such as one – compartment mode with first – order absorption and two – compartment with intravenous bolus injection, the derivatized expressions consist of more than two exponentials. We can not perform any linear transformation. Moreover, for the estimation of the disposition parameters in pharmacokinetics study, it is usual to conduct data analyses by the residual method. It is obvious that both arbitrary ignorance of contribution of the absorption to the terminal phase and log – transformation of data is responsible for inaccuracy and bias in the parameter estimation.

(2) Nonlinear Regression

Nonlinear regression has more universality. When the relationship can be defined as nonlinear model, nonlinear regression, based on the input data and functional expression (ie, algebric and differential equations), is applied to the "best fit". Determination of parameters by nonlinear regression cannot be done in a single step. Typical of least squares procedures, the fit is measured by the sum of the squares of the deviations of the observed values from the fitted values. The best fit results from an iterative procedure (also known as algorithm). An initial set of parameters is supplied by the program or by the user. The new estimates result in a better fit to the data. The procedure is repeated using the new estimates, which results in a better fit than that observed in the previous iteration. When the fit, as measured by the sum of the squares of deviations, is negligibly improved, the procedure is stopped. Iterative algorithm includes Nelder – Mead Simplex and Levenberg – Marquardt Modification (Gauss – Newton algorithm).

4. Compartmental approach in pharmacokinetics study

Pharmacokinetics is the study of kinetics of absorption, distribution, metabolism and excretion (ADME) of drugs and their corresponding pharmacologic, therapeutic, or toxic responses in man and animals. In the study, it is essential to understand the anatomy and physiology of the biologic system receiving drug as well as concepts and limitations in the model. Models used for characterization of drug exposure – time are mainly classified as compartmental model and physiologic model. The former was earlier recognized and utilized. Compartmental approach allow the definition of the relationship between the amount (or level) of drug and time by virtue of Chemical Kineitcs theory and compartment conceptualization. The most frequently used compartmental models such one – and two – compartment models are listed as follows

MODEL 1. One–compartment open model, Ⅳ injection.

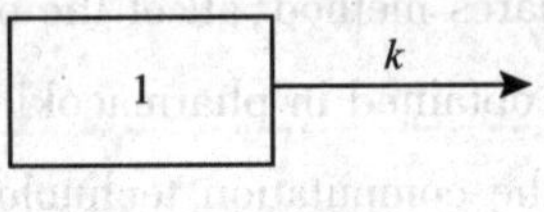

MODEL 2. One–compartment open model with first–order absorption.

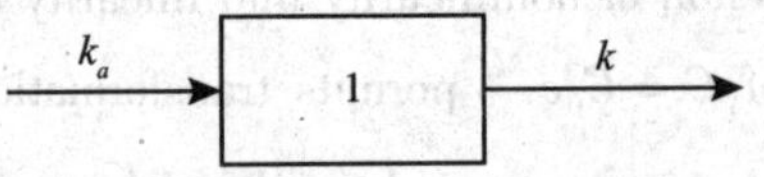

MODEL 3. Two–compartment open model, Ⅳ injection.

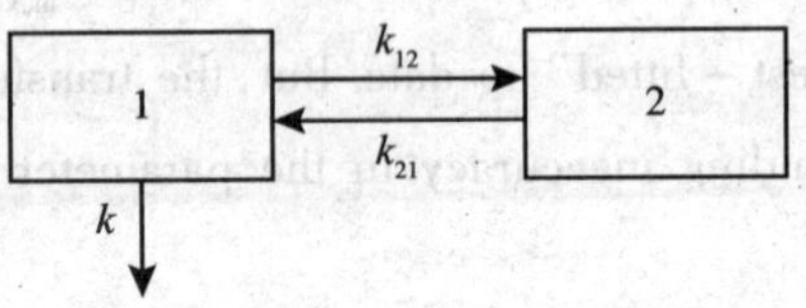

MODEL 4. Two–compartment open model with first–order absorption.

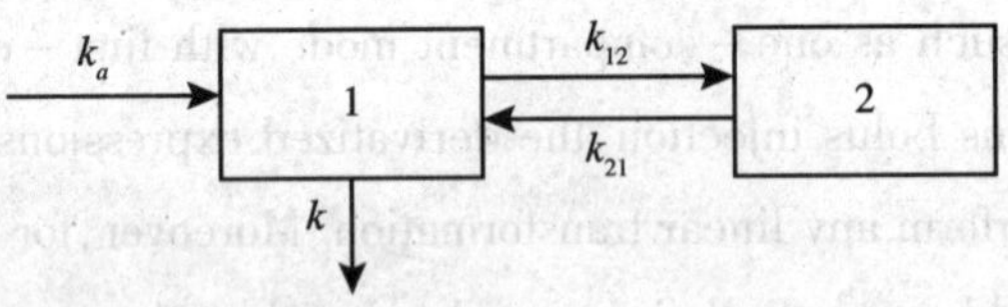

The corresponding equations defining the relationship between the drug concentration and the time are listed below.

$$C = \frac{X_0}{V_d} e^{-kt} \tag{9-2}$$

$$C = \frac{k_a F X_0}{V_d (k_a - k)} (e^{-kt} - e^{-k_a t}) \tag{9-3}$$

$$C = Ae^{-\alpha t} + Be^{-\beta t} \tag{9-4}$$

$$C = Ne^{-k_a t} + Le^{-\alpha t} + Me^{-\beta t} \tag{9-5}$$

5. Model selection

(1) Graphic visual inspection

It a plot of log concentration versus time visually indicates linearity for data obtained following intravous bolous injection, one – compartment model might appear. Otherwise, multi – compartment model occurs. But, this approach is highly associated with arbitrary judgement and biasness.

(2) Statistics metrics

a. Sum of squares of the residuals (SS)

$$SS = \sum_{i=1}^{n} (Y_i - Y_i^*)^2 \quad (9-6)$$

b. Coefficient of determination (R^2)

$$R^2 = 1 - \frac{\sum_{i=1}^{n} (Y_i - Y_i^*)^2}{\sum_{i=1}^{n} Y_i^2} \quad (9-7)$$

c. the Akaike's Information Criterion (AIC)

$$AIC = N \cdot \ln(SS) + 2M \quad (9-8)$$

Where SS is Sum of squares of the residuals, N is the number of data groups, and M is the number of parameters in the defined function.

In model selection, less the magnitude of SS and AIC, better the goodness – of – fit, and closer the fitted data to thereal ones. But the selection criteria for the better model is AIC, taking into account of the number of parameters involved.

Procedures

1. Introduction of the computer programs including software 3p97 and the damonstration
2. Nonlinear regression in the pharmacokinetic data fitting

Question 1. One patient was intravenously given of 100mg of drug A. Plasam drug A concentrations were assayed and listed in Table 9 – 1.

Tab. 9 – 1　Pharmacokinetic data of drug A (Ⅳ)

T(hours)	0.25	0.5	0.75	1.0	1.25	1.5	2	3	4
C(mg/ml)	58.98	54.10	49.59	46.65	43.38	41.02	36.73	30.58	26.54
T(hours)	6	8	10	12	16	20	24	36	48
C(mg/ml)	22.20	19.23	17.41	15.59	12.71	10.36	8.45	4.57	2.48

Question 2. One patient was intravenously given of 100mg of drug B. Plasam drug B concentrations were assayed and listed in Table 9 – 2.

Tab. 9 – 2　Pharmacokinetic data of drug B (Ⅳ)

T(hours)	0.25	0.5	0.75	1.0	2.0	3.0	4.0	6.0	8.0	10.0	14	18	24
C(mg/ml)	11.62	10.31	10.96	9.70	9.55	7.65	7.45	5.34	4.70	3.43	2.29	1.30	0.71

Question 3. One patient orally received 100mg of given antibiotic drug. Plasam drug concentrations were assayed and listed in Table 9 – 3

Tab. 9 – 3　Pharmacokinetic date of drug B (Po)

T(hours)	0.2	0.4	0.6	0.8	1.0	1.5	2.5	4.0	5.0	6.0	7.0
C(mg/ml)	1.65	2.33	2.55	2.51	2.40	2.00	1.27	0.66	0.39	0.25	0.15

Questions

1. In pharmacokinetic modeling, what is main disadvantage in the application of the residual method?

2. What kind of regression is applied in the residual method?

3. In model selection, what are routine indices proving goodness of fit? Which one is of most significance?

4. If compared to SS in the model selection, why is AIC more important?

References

1. Bourne D. *Mathematical Modeling of Pharmacokinetic Data*[M]. Lancaster, PA: Technomic Publishing, 1995.

2. Gibaldi M. *Biopharmaceutics and Clinical Pharmacokinetics*. 3rd ed[M]. Philadelphia, PA: Lea and Febiger, 1984.

3. Jambhekar S and Breen PJ. *Basic Pharmacokinetics*. 2nd ed[M]. Philadelphia, PA: Pharmaceutical Press, 2012.

4. Bonate PL. *Pharmacokinetic – Pharmacodynamic Modeling and Simulation*[M]. New York, NY: Springer, 2006.

实验十　生物等效性分析

扫码“学一学”

【目的与要求】

1. **掌握**　3p97 计算机程序在生物等效性分析中的应用。
2. **了解**　生物等效性基本概念和生物等效性分析方法。

【基本概念和实验原理】

生物等效性是指含有相同药物、相同摩尔剂量的试验制剂与参比标准制剂在类似试验条件下，两者生物利用度无统计差别或具有统计学可比性。通过研究试验制剂的生物等效性，可预期这两种制剂的临床疗效、不良反应甚至毒性可比性。药物制剂生物等效性已经成为国内外药物仿制或移植品种的重要评价指标，是药物制剂研究与开发中的重要内容之一。

在研究制剂生物等效性时，通常要分析的参数是血药浓度 - 时间曲线下面积（AUC），峰浓度（$C_{\max}$）和峰时（T_{p}），其中 AUC 是最重要的参数。即使口服给药后两种制剂具有相同的 AUC，如果由于不同的吸收速度而有不同的 $C_{\max}$ 和 T_{p}，亦不能认为具有生物等效性，但是如果吸收速度差别是设计目标且在药品说明书上如实表示，或者此差别对药品安全性和有效性无至关重要的作用的话，只要吸收程度无差别，可认为具有生物等效性。

对于许多药物制剂而言，人们会认为这些参数 20% 的差别具有临床意义。然而，对一些药物来税，这些参数的统计学显著性差别可能并不一定意味临床上的显著差别。FDA 制定的制剂生物等效性标准是：供试制剂与参比制剂的 AUC 对数比值的 90% 可信限在 0. 80 ~ 1. 25 置信区间内；供试制剂与参比制剂的 $C_{\max}$ 对数比值的 90% 可信限在 0. 70 ~ 1. 43 置信区间内；供试制剂与参比制剂的 AUC、$C_{\max}$ 的双向单侧 t 检验均得到 $p<0.05$ 的结果，T_{p} 经非参数法检验无差异。如分析成立的话，则供试制剂与参比制剂具有生物等效性，两者为生物等效性制剂。从而可做为药品监督管理部门的决策依据。

所采用的统计学方法应具有足够的灵敏度，能保证发现与个体差别无关的吸收程度和速度差别。具体的统计分析方法如下。

1. 方差分析　是常用的组间差异检验的显著性检验方法，用于评价受试制剂组和参比制剂组的组内和组间差异，即个体间、试验周期间、制剂间的差异。该法也是其它统计分析方法的基础。方差分析中通常将把握度（1 - a）设为 80%，a = 0. 2，显著性水平为 0. 5。

2. 90%置信区间分析　按下式计算供试制剂与参比制剂参数的 90% 置信区间对数值：

$$(\overline{X}_T - \overline{X}_R) \pm t_{0.1(v)} \times s\sqrt{2/n} \qquad (10-1)$$

式中，$t_{0.1(v)}$ 有 t 值表查得，计算值取反对数即为供试制剂与参比制剂参数比值的 90% 置信区间

3. 双单侧 t 检验法　进行等效性检验是国际上通行的标准方法，其他方法虽可使用，但均以双单侧 t 检验法结果为准。

双单侧 t 检验法的假设为：

无效假设 H_0：

$$\overline{X}_T - \overline{X}_R \leqslant \ln r_1 \quad (10-2)$$

$$\overline{X}_T - \overline{X}_R \geqslant \ln r_2 \quad (10-3)$$

备选假设 H_1：

$$\overline{X}_T - \overline{X}_R > \ln r_1 \quad (10-4)$$

$$\overline{X}_T - \overline{X}_R < \ln r_2 \quad (10-5)$$

检验统计量：

$$t_1 = [(\overline{X}_T - \overline{X}_R) - \ln r_1] \Big/ \left(\sqrt{\frac{2s^2}{n}}\right) \quad (10-6)$$

$$t_2 = [\ln r_2 - (\overline{X}_T - \overline{X}_R)] \Big/ \left(\sqrt{\frac{2s^2}{n}}\right) \quad (10-7)$$

式中，$\overline{X}_T$ 和$\overline{X}_R$ 分别为供试制剂与参比制剂的 *AUC* 或 $C_{\max}$ 的对数均值（原始数据经对数转换）；当检验参数为经对数转换的 *AUC* 时，r_1和 r_2分别为 0.8 和 1.25；当检验参数为经对数转换的 $C_{\max}$时，r_1和 r_2分别为 0.7 和 1.43；s 为来自方差分析的样本误差均方的平方根，n 为样本数。按假设检验理论，t_1与 t_2均服从自由度为 n－2 的 t 分布，临界值 $t_{1-\alpha}(v)$ 可由 t 单侧分位数表得到，当 $t_1 \geqslant t_{1-\alpha}(v)$ 与 $t_2 \geqslant t_{1-\alpha}(v)$ 同时成立，则拒绝 H_0，接受 H_1，认为制剂间生物等效。

【实验内容】

一、3p97 程序介绍

二、数据处理

应用 3p97 程序处理以下数据，并列出相应的统计判断依据。

例 1　剂量相等的某试验制剂 T 以参比制剂 R 为对照进行人体生物利用度实验，测得 12 名受试者的 $AUC^{0-\infty}$（表 10－1）。如仅以 *AUC* 为生物等效性分析参数，试分析试验制剂 T 与标准参比制剂 R 是否生物等效性，将分析结果填入表 10－3。

表 10－1　服用试验制剂 T 和参比制剂 R 后人体血药浓度曲线下面积

受试者	试验制剂 T		标准参比制剂 R	
	周期	$AUC^{0-\infty}$ (h×mg/ml)	周期	$AUC^{0-\infty}$ (h×mg/ml)
1	1	290	2	210
2	2	201	1	163
3	1	187	2	116
4	1	168	2	77
5	2	200	1	220
6	2	151	1	133
7	1	294	2	140
8	2	97	1	190
9	2	228	1	168
10	1	250	2	161
11	1	293	2	240
12	2	154	1	188

例 2　试验制剂 T 和参比制剂 R 进行人体生物利用度实验，受试者人数为 10 人，剂量相等，单剂量交叉给药后测得 $AUC^{0-\infty}$（表 10－2）。试分析两制剂是否具有生物等效性，将分析结果填入表 10－3。

表 10－2　试验制剂 T 和参比制剂 R 人体血药浓度曲线下面积

受试者	试验制剂 T		参比制剂 R	
	周期	$AUC^{0-\infty}$（h × mg/ml）	周期	$AUC^{0-\infty}$（h × mg/ml）
1	1	26.89	2	34.01
2	2	29.30	1	33.93
3	2	43.83	1	36.16
4	1	27.82	2	24.26
5	1	31.53	2	29.48
6	2	31.51	1	32.87
7	2	30.24	1	28.00
8	1	33.08	2	33.02
9	1	26.39	2	27.53
10	2	28.40	1	28.50

表 10－3　生物等效性分析简表

参数	试验制剂 T	参比制剂 R	T/R 比值（%）	90% 置信区间	T *vs* R 方差分析	T *vs* R 把握度
例 1 $AUC^{0-\infty}$						
例 2 $AUC^{0-\infty}$						

【实验指导】

一、预习要求

了解　生物等效性的基本概念和评价方法；双单侧 t 检验和方差分析的原理和方法。

二、思考题

1. 生物等效性在新药研究和开发中的作用和意义是什么？
2. 常用的生物等效性统计分析方法有哪些？
3. 为什么把 AUC 的等效性分析的置信区间定为 80% ~125%？

扫码“练一练”

参考文献

1. 梁文权．生物药剂学与药物动力学，［M］2 版．北京：人民卫生出版社，2004.

2. 魏树礼．生物药剂学与药物动力学［M］．北京：北京医科大学、中国协和医科大学联合出版社，1997.

3. Leon Shargel and Andrew Yu. Applied Biopharmaceutics & Pharmacokinetics. 4th ed. Stamford，Connecticut，USA，Appleton & Lange，1999

Experiment 10 Bioequivalence Assessment

Purposes

1. To acquire the experience in the use of the computer program 3p97 in the evaluation of bioequivalence.

2. To understand the concept of bioequivalence and the method for the evaluation of bioequivalence.

Introduction

Bioequivalence indicates statistically comparable bioavailability of a drug with pharmaceutical equivalents at the same molar dose under similar experimental conditions. The same bioavailability after oral administration of two different formulations implies the same extent as well the same rate of absorption. Assessment of bioequivalence might ensure the comparability of clinical therapeutic effects, side effects and even toxic effects of these drug products. It is one of important criteria used in the evaluation of the generic products all over the world.

Presently, the pharmacokinetic parameters required for the evaluation of bioequivalence are *AUC* (the area under plasma drug level – time curve from time zero to *t* or infinity), C_{max} (peak concentration) and T_p (time to reaches C_{max}), which define the systemic exposure profile. *AUC* has been regarded as the most important parameter. Even if two different formulations produce the same *AUC* after oral administration, bioequivalence does not exist if the concentration – time profiles such as C_{max} and T_p are different from each other owing to the different rates of absorption. A drug product that differs from the reference product in its rate of absorption, but not in its extent of absorption, may be considered bioequivalent if the difference in the rate of absorption is intentional and appropriately reflected in the proposed labeling and/or the rate of absorption is not detrimental to the safety and effectiveness of the drug product.

For many drug products, a ±20% difference is considered clinically important. However, a statistically significant difference between the parameter values may not necessarily represent a clinically significant difference for some drugs. In 1977, FDA has carefully established percent differences between products as ±20%, depending on the particular drug and a knowledge of the clinical relevance of drug.

The requirements to determine bioequivalence of the test (generic) drug product to the reference product include:

(1) The 90% confidence limits for *AUC* ratio of the test product to reference product, based on log transformation of the data, are within the 0.80 to 1.25 (80% ~ 125%).

(2) The 90% confidence limits for C_{max} ratio of the test product to reference product, based on log transformation of the data, are within the 0.70 to 1.143 (80% ~ 134%).

(3) In addition, two one – sided statistical tests of *AUC* and C_{max} of the test and reference products should demonstrate the confidence interval at the significance level of 5% ($p < 0.05$) using log – transformed data. Nonparameteric tests should also demonstrate no difference between the mean

T_p s of the test and reference products.

If the results of these statistical tests comply with the criteria, the test and reference products are said to be bioequivalent. Therefore, it provides the related government regulatory agency with the proofs in approving the marketing entry of the generic product. In addition, the statistical techniques used should be of sufficient sensitivity to detect differences in the rate and extent of absorption that are not attributable to subject variability.

The practical approaches for the evaluation of bioequivalence include:

(1) Crossover design

The crossover study design is utilized inbioequivalence evaluation. In this design, volunteers are once again randomly assigned to two groups, but each group receives all the treatments in the study. Hence, every volunteer will receive both the test and reference product. The washout mentioned, a predetermined period of time between the two treatment periods, is intended to prevent any carryover of effects from the first treatment to the second treatment period.

(2) Estimation of 90% confidence intervals (90% CIs)

The confidence interval is a function of sample size, and study design, including inter – and intra – subject variability. Currently, the FAD recommendations use a 90% confidence interval (CIs) (a = 0.10). The actual calculation of the 90% confidence interval would be:

$$(\overline{X}_T - \overline{X}_R) \pm t_{0.1(v)} \times s\sqrt{2/n} \qquad (10-1)$$

$t_{0.1(v)}$ abeve can be obtained by referring to value table, antilog of calculated value is 90% confiderce intervals for the parameters ratio of test preparation and reference preparation.

(3) Two one – sided statistical tests

Two one – sided statistical tests are standard methods utilized in equivalence evaluation. Although other methods can be utilized, results of two one – sided statistical test would be taken preferably.

If the tests are used, the hypotheses would be:

Null hypothesis (H_o):

$$\overline{X}_T - \overline{X}_R \leqslant \ln r_1 \qquad (10-2)$$

$$\overline{X}_T - \overline{X}_R \geqslant \ln r_2 \qquad (10-3)$$

Alternative hypothesis (H_1):

$$\overline{X}_T - \overline{X}_R > \ln r_1 \qquad (10-4)$$

$$\overline{X}_T - \overline{X}_R < \ln r_2 \qquad (10-5)$$

Statistical results:

$$t_1 = [(\overline{X}_T - \overline{X}_R) - \ln r_1] / \left(\sqrt{\frac{2s^2}{n}}\right) \qquad (10-6)$$

$$t_2 = [\ln r_2 - (\overline{X}_T - \overline{X}_R)] / \left(\sqrt{\frac{2s^2}{n}}\right) \qquad (10-7)$$

where $\overline{X}_T$ and $\overline{X}_R$ are the means of logarithm – transformed *AUC* and/or C_{max} of the test and reference product, respectively. *s* is the pooled variance in ANOVA. *n* is the sample size per level of the discrete independent variable. When log – transformed AUC is involved, r_1 and r_2 are 0.8 and 1.25, respectively. And when log – transformed C_{max} is involved, r_1 and r_2 are 0.7 and 1.43, respectively.

In this case, we deal with two null hypotheses which indicate outcomes outside of the acceptable differences for bioequivalence. The two alternative hypotheses represent outcomes that fall short of the extremes. If both $t_1 \geqslant t_{1-\alpha}(v)$ and $t_2 \geqslant t_{1-\alpha}(v)$ apply, H_0 is rejected and H_1 is accepted. As a result, it is concluded that the test (generic) and the reference products are said to be bioequivalent drug products.

Procedures

1. Introduction and demonstration of the application of the computer program 3p97.
2. Application of 3p97 in the following cases for the evaluation of bioequivalence.

Example 1. In the study for assessing bioequivalence, the test (T) and reference (R) products of the same molar doses were orally given to 12 healthy volunteers. Perform the related statistical tests in order to determine bioequivalence of the test product to the reference only using the estimated *AUC*s in Tab. 10 – 1 and fill the results in Tab. 10 – 3.

Tab. 10 – 1 The estimated $AUC^{0-\infty}$ in a bioequivalence study of two drug products in 12 human volunteers

Subjects	T		R	
	Study period	$AUC^{0-\infty}$ (h ×mg/ml)	Study period	$AUC^{0-\infty}$ (h ×mg/ml)
1	1	290	2	210
2	2	201	1	163
3	1	187	2	116
4	1	168	2	77
5	2	200	1	220
6	2	151	1	133
7	1	294	2	140
8	2	97	1	190
9	2	228	1	168
10	1	250	2	161
11	1	293	2	240
12	2	154	1	188

Example 2. In the study for assessing bioequivalence, the test (T) and reference (R) products of the same molar doses were orally given to 10 healthy volunteers. Perform the related statistical tests in order to determine bioequivalence of the test product to the reference only using the estimated *AUC*s in Tab. 10 – 2 and fill the results in Tab. 10 – 3.

Tab. 10 – 2 The estimated $AUC^{0-\infty}$ in a bioequivalence study of two drug products in 10 human volunteers

Subjects	T		R	
	Study period	$AUC^{0-\infty}$ (h × mg/ml)	Study period	$AUC^{0-\infty}$ (h × mg/ml)
1	1	26.89	2	34.01
2	2	29.30	1	33.93

continued

Subjects	T		R	
	Study period	$AUC^{0-\infty}$ (h×mg/ml)	Study period	$AUC^{0-\infty}$ (h×mg/ml)
3	2	43.83	1	36.16
4	1	27.82	2	24.26
5	1	31.53	2	29.48
6	2	31.51	1	32.87
7	2	30.24	1	28.00
8	1	33.08	2	33.02
9	1	26.39	2	27.53
10	2	28.40	1	28.50

Tab. 10-3 Bioavailability comparison of a test and reference products in the bioequivalence assessment

Parameters	T (AVG ± SD)	R (AVG ± SD)	T/R Ratio(%)	90% Confidence Limits	T vs R ANOVA	T vs R Power test
$AUC^{0-\infty}$ in Case 1						
$AUC^{0-\infty}$ in Case 2						

Experimental Guidelines

Requirements for preview

(1) To understand the methods and concepts in the assessment of bioequivalene.

(2) To be well prepared with a knowledge of the related computer softwares.

Questions

(1) To discuss the significance of bioequivalence in the development of the drug products.

(2) To review the common methods necessary for the assessment of bioequivalence.

(3) To explain why the confidence interval is set at 0.80 to 1.25 in the assessment ofbioequivalence

References

1. Liang Wen Quan. Biopharmaceutics and Pharmacokinetics. 2nd edition [M]. Beijing: The People's Sanitation Publishing Company. 2004.

2. Wei Shu Li. Biopharmaceutics and Pharmacokinetics [M]. Beijing: United Publishing Press of Beijing Medical University and China Peking Union University. 1997.

3. Leon Shargel and Andrew Yu. Applied Biopharmaceutics & Pharmacokinetics. 4th ed. Stamford, Connecticut, USA, Appleton & Lange, 1999.